Health and Medicine
in the Jewish Tradition

Health/Medicine and the Faith Traditions

Edited by Martin E. Marty and Kenneth L. Vaux

Health/Medicine and the Faith Traditions
explores the ways in which major religions
relate to the questions of human well-being.
It issues from Project Ten, an interfaith program
of The Park Ridge Center, An Institute for the Study of
Health, Faith, and Ethics.

James P. Wind, Director of Research and Publications

The Park Ridge Center,
a Division of the Lutheran Institute of Human Ecology,
is part of the Lutheran General Health Care System,
in Park Ridge, Illinois.

Health
and Medicine
in the Jewish
Tradition

L'HAYYIM—TO LIFE

David M. Feldman

Crossroad · New York

1986
The Crossroad Publishing Company
370 Lexington Ave, New York, N.Y. 10017

Library of Congress Cataloging in Publication Data
Feldman, David M.
Health and medicine in the Jewish tradition.
1. Health—Religious aspects—Judaism.
2. Medicine—Religious aspects—Judaism.   3. Marriage—
Religious aspects—Judaism.   4. Abortion—Religious
aspects—Judaism.   5. Medical ethics.   I. Title.
[DNLM: 1. Ethics, Medical.   2. Judaism.   3. Religion
and Medicine. W 50 F312h]
BM538.H43F44   1986   296.3'85   85-29074
ISBN   0-8245-0707-X

To Aviva
and to Daniel, Jonathan and Rebecca
with love

Contents

Foreword

The books in this series in every case are for two sets of people: (a) those who are in the tradition being discussed and (b) everyone else. The editors assume that readers who are somehow in a tradition will bring one set of curiosities. They may simply wish to be informed, to gain something of an intellectual character about the religious past that somehow shapes them now. Or they may wish to clarify their own attitudes toward elements of the tradition and put these to work in their own search for health.

"Everyone else" also has good reasons for reading. In the modern world, in a pluralist society like the one from which this book issues, traditions and the people in them surround each other. They collide. They interact. They serve or can serve as catalysts. One is attended to medically by people of other traditions. People in medical professions ordinarily do not take care only of their own. If patients and professionals have resources for promoting well-being these can often be borrowed. They can also be taught to those who do not become fully at home in a tradition.

It is important to point to these two readerships in every case. In no instance, however, is it likely to be as urgent as in the case of Judaism. At first glance, Judaism seems to be quite small. The *Encyclopaedia Britannica Yearbook* for 1984 listed only 17,320,140 Jews in the world, with 7,611,940 of these in North America. A single, albeit the largest, American Protestant denomination, the Southern Baptist Convention, which does not include small children in its numbering, listed 13,782,644 members in a 1983 yearbook. All this statistical talk may seem to be beside the point, yet it helps promote the main point. On the world scale of religions, Judaism, alongside a billion Christians and a half billion Muslims, is very tiny, hardly noticeable. Yet, on the world scale of religious influence, especially in respect to health and medicine, Judaism is very large, never ignorable.

Professor Feldman does not spend too much time saying exactly why Judaism has such influence on its own people and on others. He hurries right to the point, his point being a thematic development of inherited Jewish concerns about well-being through all the cycles of life. Yet it is valid for us to linger for a moment in the waiting room and get a sense of the environment in respect to this topic. Why does Judaism loom so large and have so much to say?

The first reason, and this begins to become clear in the Feldman treatment, is textual. The Hebrew Scriptures, which stand behind many Jewish motifs, bear a tradition which has shaped a distinctive and remarkable people. This tradition spills over any barriers of peoplehood; witness how its history and ideas have been taken over as the "Old Testament" by Christians. This taking over does violence to these Scriptures as Jews read them. They make Judaism a script for a two-act drama in which it plays a role Jews do not accept in the unfolding of the second act. Yet that act of violence is bonded with acts of devotion. Christians, the vast majority in North America and the people who make up the largest of the world religions, share a story, a covenant, a set of ways of life, practices, and habits from Jews. Islam, which in the eyes of Jews does even more violence to the Hebrew Scriptures, also reworks but shares the story and can never simply extricate itself from its bonds with Israel. Whatever else the Scriptures mean to Jews, and they do not mean everything—the Feldman treatment of rabbinic texts makes that clear—these are a point of connection far beyond Judaism.

A second reason for attention to Jewish views of health, medicine, illness, and well-being is to be associated with the recent past, the historical record of Judaism. Jews, despised and persecuted as they have often been, and full of problems of their own in respect to their religious heritage, have helped set the pace in the development of modern medicine. At one point David Feldman's book seems to have been torn from the phonebook or a medical *Who's Who* as he prints a register of pioneers who were Jews. That way of putting it suggests a problem: Were these physicians and scientists acting out of the Jewish tradition, or did their interest in medicine displace or replace the religious element of their heritage? Did they, to use the modern phrase so unfair to historic faith, just "happen to be Jews"? No doubt something of all of these possibilities went into the outcome, yet it is hard to picture modern, often at least semisecular and sometimes frankly nonreligious Jews uninfluenced by the lore they acquired from their ancestors in the faith.

While readers ponder the possible explanations, they do well at least to notice the connections between Jews and Judaism and medicine. Jewish humorists often suggest that being a doctor "goes with the territory" for bright young Jews: "My son the doctor . . ." is the first line of many a joke. In many communities there is a Jewish hospital, sometimes a legacy of a time when others would not accept Jews and just as often an expression of Jewish responsibility for its city. Social scientists in the field of medicine like to observe Jewish practices and their impact on health: Are they more or less devoted to alcohol, more or less prone to mental illness? Jews make up the core of much social and cultural philanthropy. Their tradition impels them to help assure medical research, the building of hospitals and universities. From Sigmund Freud through David Bakan, students of the psyche and therapists have drawn on Jewish story—of "Moses and Monotheism," of Job, and more—to inform contemporary inquiry. The story of medicine minus Judaism would be significantly shorter and poorer.

Professor Feldman sketches many reasons for the Jewish concern with well-being. It is essentially a this-worldly faith, one that expects ethical response in this world more than salvation in one to come. From the first, there have been preoccupations with behavior in spheres where illness or health might result; witness the discussion of circumcision and the laws and rites when the health of a baby is at stake. Witness also the concern over menstruation, care of the body, attention to the needs of the dying in the Judaism outlined on these pages.

To protect Professor Feldman and aid the reader, it may be important to note that no one can speak out of all of Judaism for all of Judaism to the satisfaction of all heirs of Judaism. Even Roman Catholicism, which centers its teaching authority in the pope, cannot produce agreed-upon treatments of topics like this. Certainly Protestantism, with its hundreds of denominations, could not produce a single work that would satisfy all. Judaism stands somewhere between these extremes, for it is denominationalized in America, full of contention elsewhere, not simply chaotic, but by no means unified. A book by an Orthodox rabbi would be more uncompromising in its depiction of observances, while a Reform advocate would write out of the experience of a lineage that, in Europe and America, has attempted to remain faithful to what is Jewish while reaching as far as possible to anticipate new circumstances.

Professor Feldman comes from the Conservative tradition, which would be treated unfairly if it were characterized as "half way between," a compromise that must tolerate extremes. Instead, this movement represents a very conscious choice to seek fidelity to the Jewish tradition on one hand and to express a dynamic or developmental character in relation to modernity on the other. Where it adapts, it does so not because it has no choice but because it chooses to think that is what Judaism must do. In some respects, the Orthodox and Reform movements aspire to do the same. Yet a one-author book can only be by one author, and in choosing Feldman out of Conservatism we feel we have not rejected the many credible candidates out of others, but have presented someone who, on his own, is in touch with sacred writings of this tradition and alert to developments in the world he, and we all, must inhabit.

Writers of forewords are supposed to help locate the books they introduce, not to take away the suspense such book plots have to build to make their case. I resist commenting on the substance of Feldman's treatment. A final service, then, might result from an attempt to describe the genre. Some volumes in this series include straightforward historical narrative. Some are sustained ethical treatises. While one will have a therapeutic intention, another might suggest the role of the diagnostician or observer. In the present case, Feldman combines commentary on Jewish texts ancient and modern with anecdotes and rabbinic stories. This is not an idiosyncracy: It has roots in ancient and enduring Jewish modes. The author takes up a theme, illustrates it from the Jewish past, tells what the rabbis had to say, jumps with ease to modern instances, and engages in reflection—before moving on to another of the topics that preoccupy all the writers in this series. The medium and the message are linked in this method. This is not the only way Jews reason in respect to the search for human well-being. Yet this is faithful to one of the main modes, and is likely to draw and hold the attention of many for whom the detailed history is simply too detailed. They would leave that to professional historians. It can appeal to those who believe that "Jewish theology" is an uncongenial category for a faith that is really a history, or a way. Yes, that is it: This is a book, illustrated from a long tradition, of the Jewish "way." It has much to say to inform and help (a) Jews and (b) everybody else.

MARTIN E. MARTY
The University of Chicago

Preface

This book makes its appearance in response to the specific summons by the creators of Project Ten, and to the general need for considering the Jewish tradition on matters of health and medicine. Old questions and new possibilities have raised consciousness about ethical and religious concerns in this area, concerns addressed by the Jewish tradition with both classic authority and compelling wisdom.

The repository of this tradition begins with the Bible, which is the common property of and accessible to most of the world, and continues through a literary heritage essentially unavailable in translation—Talmud and its commentaries, moral and philosophic tracts, and codes of law. These are refracted in the voluminous Responsa literature that refines the legal-moral tradition and gives it its contemporary application and implications.

The present work offers a brief overview of its subject in the light of the historic faith tradition of Judaism. It sets forth the precepts affirmed and the stance taken, the principles and the value system reflected. The scope of the overview is, of course, defined by the parameters of this series and is designed in conformity with its concise but highly relevant perspective. As to mode of presentation, empirical and anecdotal narrative are offered alongside the relay of theoretical or objective doctrine.

Elements of the book's fundamental thesis will nonetheless emerge with adequate clarity: that in Jewish law and practice the pursuit of preventive and curative medicine is held in high esteem and, rather than a theological problem, is a religious obligation; that human life is to be revered for its own sake, above conflicting ritual demands, on the one hand, or its apparent lack of quality, on the other; that health implies a respectful concern for body and soul, unhyphenated; and that these objectives are to be sought in the individual, social, sexual and therapeutic dimensions of life.

"*L'Hayyim*—To Life" is the book's subtitle, epitomizing Judaism's joyous affirmation of this-worldly life and well-being. To do so responsibly is to fulfill God's command for one's self and for others, in the face of all challenges, human and natural.

I am grateful to the Lutheran Institute of Human Ecology for the call to prepare this volume; to the Medical Ethics Committee of New York's Federation of Jewish Philanthropies where, as chairman, I was able to explore and expound in the company of learned colleagues. I thank the officers and membership of my beloved congregation, the Jewish Center of Teaneck, who encouraged my efforts despite a heavy schedule of active ministry.

I am grateful, too, to my teachers and forebears, devoted guardians of the tradition, who have nurtured and advanced its ennobling instruction. May this proffered treatise do a measure of justice to their faith commitment and bring healing insight to the questing reader.

DAVID M. FELDMAN
Teaneck, New Jersey

· 1 ·

The Mandate to Heal

Health is clearly a desideratum, buttressed by principles and provisions of Bible and Talmud. And the Jewish people is proud of its medical practitioners, of the historic love affair between medicine and Judaism, and of the skill and compassion mandated by the Tradition and implemented by its followers. To maintain the body as well as the soul in good health is a religious imperative; to do so reflects Judaic teachings concerning body-and-soul and other theological issues, which have contributed to the role of Judaism and Jewish physicians in medicine and medical ethics.

A basic formulation of part of this attitude is found in the words of Maimonides, the famous rabbi-physician of the twelfth century, who saw fit to include hygienic recommendations in his summary, not of moral philosophy, but of the code of Jewish law: "One should aim to maintain physical health and vigor in order that his soul may be upright, in order to know God.... Whoever follows this course will be continually serving God...."[1]

Yet this religious affirmation merely serves to underscore the implied philosophic problems. There is a desire to be well, even a religious obligation to do so. But does healing, or sickness for that matter, come from God or from man? May we intervene in God's scheme of things and add our healing efforts to what He and He alone can do? That would seem to betray a lack of faith in God as healer. More to the point, may we *contravene* God's scheme of things and heal when He has made ill, thwart His apparent purpose by removing what He has seen fit to inflict? The questions have a long history in Jewish thought.

The problem of simple intervention is addressed in the Midrash:

Rabbi Ishmael and Rabbi Akiva were walking through the streets of Jerusalem and met a sick man who asked them: "How can I be cured?" They answered: "Do thus and so until you are cured." He said to them: "But who afflicted me?" "The Holy One, blessed be He," they answered.

"So how can you interfere in a matter which is not your concern? God afflicted me and you wish to heal?" The rabbis then asked: "What is your vocation?" "I am a tiller of the soil. Here is the vine-cutter in my hand." They asked: "But who created the vineyard?" "The Holy One, blessed be He." "Well, you interfered in the vineyard which is not yours. He created it and you cut away its fruits?" they asked. "But were I not to plow and till and fertilize and weed, the vineyard would not produce any fruit," he explained. "So," they responded, "from your own work have you not learned what is written (Ps. 103:15): 'As for man, his days are as grass.' Just as the tree, if not weeded, fertilized, and plowed, will not grow and bring forth its fruits, so with the human body. The fertilizer is the medicine and the means of healing, and the tiller of the earth is the physician."[2]

Fine. Human effort is essential; we are partners in the process and we may and must intervene. But the real problem is, how can we contravene? In the words of Rashi, we might well ask, "How is it that God smites and man heals?"

Rashi's rhetorical question is asked in the context of the given answer to this problem. He is expounding the talmudic passage that bases the answer on the Bible (Ex. 21:19). There the subject is torts, damages done by one person to another. The Bible prescribes compensation to the victim by the perpetrator, including medical costs: "He must compensate for forced idleness and see that the victim is 'thoroughly healed' (*rappo y'rappei*)." "From here [from this verse we derive]," says the Talmud, "that the physician is granted permission to heal." He needs permission. Specific authorization is necessary to assure us that medical intervention is allowable.

Broader scope for the authorization comes from another talmudic passage, one chosen as the focus by Maimonides. There, in Deuteronomy 22:2, the context is the mitzvah of restoring lost objects: "If you chance upon an object lost by your brother, you must restore it to him." The Talmud (*Sanhedrin* 73a) expands the mitzvah to include rescuing a neighbor from danger, such as drowning or being attacked by an animal—that is, to "restore" his body as well as his belongings. To Maimonides, this is the biblical source of the mandate to heal: to come to the aid of one who has lost his health and needs restoration.[3] To Maimonides, the permission is implied; here we are given a commandment to heal, even implying an obligation on the part of the physician to render professional services when needed.

Not so simple, says an older contemporary of Maimonides, the Bible commentator Rabbi Abraham ibn Ezra (d. 1167). He points to a narrative in 2 Chronicles 16:12 where we are told that Asa, King of Judea, became severely ill and "sought not the Lord but the physicians." This can be understood either as censure for seeking medical help without prayer as well, or for forgetting that physicians are vehicles for God's help. But Ibn Ezra sees it as censure for seeking medical assistance at all, for not trusting in God without medicine. Ibn Ezra therefore postulates a contradiction between this passage and the Exodus one above. He resolves the difference by finding the latter to refer, as does its context, to man-made wounds, which the perpetrator must undo, and the former passage to refer to "internal wounds," sickness, which is an 'act of God.' These are presumed to be manifestations of divine rebuke or punishment and only God may heal or remove them.

Indeed, this point of view recommends itself when other biblical verses are considered, verses in which a connection is made between sin and affliction, and between righteousness or repentance and freedom from illness. After their liberation from Egyptian bondage, the Israelites are told (Ex. 15:26): "If you hearken to the voice of the Lord . . . and do what is right in His eyes . . . none of the diseases which I inflicted upon Egypt will I inflict upon you, for I am the Lord your Healer." Whereas, "If you fail to hearken . . . I will inflict upon you evil and faithful illnesses" (Deut. 28:58).

"Faithful illnesses?" What could that mean? The standard translations render something like "relentless illnesses." But the literal meaning of *ne-emanim*, "faithful," is the subject of an engaging comment by the Talmud in another connection. This precious nugget of commentary, which seems to have eluded more widespread citation, is best appreciated when one bears in mind the popular anecdote about the victim who wants to defraud his insurance company. The hero of this story is only mildly bruised in an automobile accident but has himself thoroughly bandaged, and hospitalized in traction, with all the appearance of having been rendered a total invalid. The insurance agent doesn't believe it at all but cannot effectively refute it. He pays the exorbitant claim but admonishes the client. "Here is your money," he says, "but I'm going to have you watched day and night, to make sure these bandages are for real wounds." "You can watch me all you want," replied the other. "You can even watch me tomorrow, when my valet comes to fetch me. He will carefully lift me into my car, drive me to the airport, tenderly lift me into the airplane, fly with me all the way to France. Then he will, with equally tender care, bring me to the shrine at Lourdes—and you will see with your own eyes what a splendid miracle will happen to me there!"

With something similar in mind, the Talmud has a serious discussion about the allurements of idolatry. Pagan worship seemed so attractive that the legislation in the Bible against idolatrous practices was refined and applied strictly by the talmudic teachers. In the discussion (*Avodah Zarah* 55a), one rabbi dared to suggest that perhaps there's "something to it"; perhaps the idolatrous rites or shrines may indeed have the effect they promise. "What about that time when so-and-so, a sick man, went to the place of idolatry in search of a cure, and came out healed?" he asked. The other rabbi's answer was clever. "That's what that strange phrase in Deuteronomy means," he said; those "evil and faithful illnesses." The illnesses are faithful. This illness, you must know, stipulated with almighty God that it would afflict the body of so-and-so on such-and-such a day at such-and-such an hour, and would *leave* him on such-and-such a day at such-and-such an hour. Now it so happened that the patient walked into that shrine on the very hour that had been stipulated for the illness to leave him. The illness momentarily "considered" reneging on the agreement and remaining longer with the patient, just so that the idolatrous shrine would not *appear* to have the power to cure. But it was "faithful"—faithful to leave him at the prearranged moment no matter who got the credit!

When the physician heals, this story suggests, it's all part of a preordained divine scheme. The elaborate skill and ministrations of health-care people, and the sophisticated means and medicaments made use of, are ultimately an expression of God's inexorable blueprint. God afflicts and man, in fulfillment of a divine imperative, heals.

Even, it seems, if the illness is inflicted as a punishment. This is better understood by considering a relevant point put in popular form by a great hasidic teacher. There is nothing on earth, according to this point of view, without its good aspect. But Rabbi Jacob Isaac of Pzhysha (d. 1814) asks, what good is there in, say, atheism? "I'll tell you. A poor man comes and asks for charity. You might say to yourself, 'Why should I give him charity? That would be interfering in some vast, eternal plan. If God made him poor, why should I interfere?' Rather, we are exhorted, be an atheist for a moment and give him the charity!"[4]

The affliction of poverty is no different from the affliction of illness, from this theological standpoint. In both cases, the ethical imperative bids us leave the theology to God and do our ethical duty. The rabbis, again in an unrelated context, express this idea by attributing a kind of weariness about it to God Himself. "If only," the Midrash has God say wistfully, "they would leave Me alone and just keep My commandments."[5]

As if to fulfill this wish, the Rabbis overwhelmingly took to the task of expounding the Torah in that spirit. The ethical imperative was found to be determinative everywhere, from helping the poor to healing the sick. God was to be imitated, not in His attribute of stern Justice but in His attribute of Mercy and Compassion.

This certainly seems to be the mandate of the Torah on the face of it. Ethical injunctions abound, all of which would be nullified were we piously to refrain from intervening or contravening what we see around us as a given. The Holiness Code of Leviticus, for example, is studded with moral and ethical duties. "Thou shalt not stand [idly] by the blood of thy brother" (Lev. 19:16) is specifically invoked by the Talmud as enjoining us to come to the rescue of a person in danger, and is cited by subsequent teachers as the source of the obligation to extend medical help. Nahmanides (d. 1270) sees a general obligation to save the life of one's fellow-man in the verse "Let thy brother live with thee" (Lev. 25:35). Better still, he locates the physician's obligation to heal in the famous "Love thy neighbor as thyself" (Lev. 19:18).

Altogether, the ethical imperative predominates. The nineteenth-century philosopher Hermann Cohen advanced the thesis, in his *Religion of Reason*, that the biblical prophets intuited and anticipated formal philosophic concepts associated with Kant and the modern understanding of religion. Their insights and preachments added up to what moderns called Ethical Monotheism as a formal system, a system that sees God as allowing and thus demanding improvement over the way things are. God is one, the Creator of both good and evil, yet inspiring us to ethical deeds.

But the logic still needs buttressing. In the eighteenth century, philosopher David Hume wanted to commit suicide. He was challenged: "God gives you life; how can you interfere with God's will and end it yourself?" To which he responded: "But then how can the physician interfere in the other direction, and restore life to one who—by God's will, apparently—is dying from illness?"

The question is essentially answerable only by the faith postulate that God favors apparent good over evil, life over death. It is a faith postulate sorely challenged by adverse experience: We witness evil—human suffering, natural disasters, a Holocaust. Yet we live by the faith affirmed in our High Holy Day liturgy: "Remember us to life, O King Who desirest life." We see God on the side of life. Even the universe evidences a fundamental hospitability to life, in that it makes life and growth possible. Though God is master of both life and death, good and evil, we are partners with Him only in the bias for life. We imitate only His attribute of mercy, and the ethical imperative moves us to advance the cause of life and health and good.

Death, too, is "good" and plays its role. "And God saw all that He had made and behold it was very good" (Gen. 1:31). "'Very good'—that includes death," says the Midrash.[6] Without the death of one generation, there would be no room or role for the next generation. Evil, too, has its place as the basis of comparison that makes good real. And sickness has its benevolent purposes, too—as chastisement, as motivation for health efforts, as restorer of value perspective.

But the good we see in evil is, for us, only after the fact. It is not for us to bring it about, no matter what good we see in it. After the fact, we justify it in our theodicies and find purpose in it. We must take care before crossing the street, and we must drive carefully and soberly. But if an accident does happen we seek to find reason for or justification of it retrospectively, and declare that "The Lord giveth and the Lord taketh away."

Illustrative is a mishnaic statement that, in isolation, sounds harsh and disproportionately severe: "For three sins, women die in childbirth. For negligence in [keeping the laws of] menstrual separation, the dough [*hallah*] offering, and lighting the Sabbath candles."[7] This judgment is cruel—to humans, but kind to God. It's a theodicy, a way of vindicating God's ways by placing responsibility on the victims. In childbirth, mortal hazard is highest and women are most vulnerable. If they succumb—as empirically we see they do—it must be because they have been somehow negligent or malfeasant in what pertains especially to them.

Contrast this statement with another talmudic passage (a Baraita, contemporaneous with the Mishnah): "Three kinds of women [for whom pregnancy could be marginally more hazardous than usual] should use a contraceptive [to prevent such hazard]"—which means that others, with greater likelihood of hazard, certainly should.[8] Whatever else this Baraita means, it clearly teaches that human measures should be taken to avoid those dangers of childbearing that are the subject of the other Mishnah. After the fact, we can make the most of God's judgment upon us. We can absolve Him or share in the blame. But before the fact, we are bidden to take every precaution to prevent any mishap, deserved or not.

Deserved or not. The permission to use contraception to prevent a hazardous pregnancy is not restricted to virtuous women. The classic permission, or mandate, to abort a pregnancy to save the mother's life is not dependent on her personal guilt or innocence in any matter large or small. Nor would medical treatment to cure illness—or infertility—be denied to one who does not "deserve" it. The issue was raised recently in connection with in-vitro fertilization. "Test-tube baby" clinics are private enterprises in the

U.S., but are supported by public funds in Canada and Britain. At a recent symposium in Toronto, one participant opposed the use of public money for this purpose since the infertility it corrects is caused by scarred tissue in the Fallopian tubes, ovaries and uterus. This pelvic inflammatory condition is the result, in large part, of venereal disease. The public need not, he argued, contribute to the relief of a situation brought about in sin. He went on to include AIDS research among the projects that ought not be supported. Not yet aware of its danger to others, he would veto the expenditure of money and effort to treat or cure AIDS, because the condition is the consequence of sin, in this case the sin of homosexual activity. On an unconscious level, this punitive sentiment is sometimes a component in one's position against abortion: Why cooperate in relieving the burden of the sinful perpetrator?

The ethical thrust of Leviticus and Deuteronomy is unconditional. Restore the lost object; uphold your faltering brother; open your hand to the poor; be kind to the stranger, the orphan, the widow; help even your enemy in trouble. All these imperatives are to be followed without fear that you may be depriving someone of his just deserts.

Or yourself. Charity begins at home; the ethical injunction points to the self as well, to take every precaution to avoid a mishap. And we are more than just bidden to prevent mishap. Avoidance of hazard, circumventing danger or even possible danger—these are elevated to the highest level of mitzvah. Preservation of life and health is a mitzvah of first rank; by permission and obligation they call for "setting aside the rest of the Torah," such as Sabbath and Yom Kippur.

For this fundamental theme, we turn to a new chapter.

· 2 ·

"Set Aside the Torah" to Protect Life and Health

The primacy of preservation of life and health is associated with three distinct biblical verses. The exegetical derivations are offered in the name of three different sages in the talmudic treatment of the subject.

"How do we know that avoidance of a threat to life sets aside the Sabbath?" asks the Talmud (*Yoma* 85b). Rabbi Simon ben Menassia: "We are told: 'You shall keep the Sabbath, for it is holy unto you' (Ex. 31:13). That means, unto *you* is the Sabbath given over, but you are not given over to the Sabbath." Rabbi Nathan: "We are told: 'The people of Israel shall keep the Sabbath, to observe the Sabbath through the generations' (Ex. 31:16). That means, violate one Sabbath if necessary in order to keep many Sabbaths afterward." Rabbi Yehudah in the name of Rabbi Samuel: "We are told: 'Keep My commandments and ordinances, which if a man do them he will live by them' (Lev. 18:5). That means, live by them and don't die because of them."

There is much to say, historically and legally, about each of these exegetical teachings. The first, where the Sabbath is given over to you rather than vice versa, was tested in practice in the days of the Maccabees (second pre-Christian century). In that first war for religious freedom, when the Judeans went to battle against the Greek Syrians in the days of Antiochus, the enemy attacked on the Sabbath on the assumption they would meet no resistance then. But, in keeping with the Talmud's teaching above, they did rise in self-defense even on the Sabbath.

Thus Jesus, too, was in good rabbinical tradition when he responded to those who objected to his healing efforts on the Sabbath. He affirmed "The Sabbath is given to man, not man to the Sabbath."[1]

The second exegetical point has implications for basic orientation to life.

Is the focus of religious efforts this world or the next? In an otherworldly orientation it would not matter much if one were to die in observing the Sabbath. His reward would be condign in the next world. But in a this-worldly attitude, the goal is to preserve life, to remain alive here on earth for the allotted time, to "stick around" and "keep many Sabbaths."

The third derivation gives us a principle and, at the same time, a statement of exceptions thereto. "Not die because of them"—except, that is, in the case of one of the three cardinal sins. Rather die, rather undergo martyrdom, than transgress the sin of murder, of idolatry or of adultery-incest. Otherwise, for all violations of the Torah, sins of commission or of omission, *ya'avor v-al yehareg*—let him transgress rather than be killed. But not for these three. If one is asked to murder (the innocent, as opposed to killing, in self-defense, a no-longer-innocent attacker), then *yehareg v-al ya'avor*, let him be killed rather than transgress the overriding commandment, "Thou shalt not murder." Or, if one is asked to bow to idols, as were Hannah and her seven sons in the days of the Maccabees, and to do so publicly, then one must accept martyrdom, as they did. Lastly, the sin of gross sexual immorality is serious enough to require martyrdom instead.

Barring these three, if observance of, say, the Sabbath or Yom Kippur or any ritual or other commandment entails a threat to one's life or health, then such a threat "sets aside the entire Torah."

Though even this seems harsh, the Talmud records it as a delimitation on martyrdom rather than a recommendation. Evidently, people were ready to martyr themselves for lesser challenges; during the Hadrianic persecutions, the rabbis, in a synod "in the upper chambers of the house of Nitza in Lydda" (*Sanhedrin* 74a) solemnly ruled that only in these situations may such extreme steps be taken.

And if this delimitation reveals, again, a this-worldly orientation, a mandate to stay alive and healthy on this earth, it also says much about the relationship between physical and spiritual well-being. As important as is proper ritual observance of Sabbath, Yom Kippur or dietary laws, they all take second place to proper care of the fundamentals of physical health. A legal principle is enunciated in the Talmud (*Hullin* 9a): *Hamira sakkanta me-issura*, "That which is [physically/medically] dangerous is worse than that which is [ritually] forbidden." Avoidance of the harmful becomes a religious precept, associated in fact with the teaching implied in the biblical verse, "Take therefore good heed of yourselves" (Deut. 4:15).[2]

This is best illustrated by the paradigmatic example of the Yom Kippur fast. As opposed to other fast days on the Jewish calendar—such as Tishah

B'Av, commemorating the destruction of the Temple in Jerusalem in 586 B.C.E. and in 70 C.E., and other rabbinically ordained fasts—Yom Kippur is biblical and the fast is fundamental to its observance. Yet, in keeping with the above, any threat to a person's health occasioned by the fast means that it becomes his mitzvah to eat rather than to abstain! The mitzvah of sustaining health overrides that of the fast, and he must eat. Of course, he is not to feast, only to take what is minimally necessary to stay in health.

What about the malingerer or the hypochondriac who only thinks he needs to eat? No such thing. In the Talmud's further discussion of the principle, the patient is supreme, the doctor second in line. "One who feels ill on Yom Kippur is fed on the advice of the physician" (*Yoma* 83a). What if the physician deems him ill but the patient feels himself strong enough to fast? We cause him to eat, because this is foolish piety. What if the physician declares him well enough to fast but the patient doesn't think so? Then we listen to the patient rather than to the doctor, as implied in scripture: "The heart knoweth its own bitterness" (Prov. 14:10). The subjective component is real. Perceived danger is also danger in this context.

The matter is summed up in the Code of Jewish Law (*Orah Hayyim* 329:3): All laws of the Torah are suspended on the possibility that life is in danger, however remote the likelihood. The Talmud, in its Palestinian recension, adds a dimension to the principle when it tells us that he who hesitates, imagining that the danger is not so great, is guilty of bloodshed if a casualty eventuates, and that even the rabbi is guilty for not having taught clearly in advance that one should not hesitate to do what is necessary in such circumstances.

A "possible threat to life" sets aside Sabbath laws and must be avoided in general, by religious precept. This means that the Sabbath should be violated to attend a woman in labor, and it means that a woman should not enter into a hazardous pregnancy. But there are normal dangers, such as ordinary pregnancy, or flying in a plane, or—smoking. What principle distinguishes these situations?

The Mishnah forbids drinking of liquids that have been left uncovered overnight, against the possibility that they may have become contaminated. It also forbids keeping a vicious dog or a faulty ladder, because of harm that might eventuate to the unwary.[3] These are in keeping with the biblical requirement (Deut. 22:8) to build a parapet or railing around the roof of a home to prevent accidental falling. Yet, when "many have accustomed themselves" to certain practices with no consequent harm, such as drinking uncovered liquids, there is the assumption of "the Lord preserves the simple." The Talmud itself (*Berakhot* 33a), in prescribing proper conduct for the Silent Prayer, allows one to break his worshipful posture and interrupt his prayer to ward off an approaching scorpion—but not a snake! The snake, commentaries explain, is quite dangerous *if* it bites, but it may not bite; while the scorpion more likely will. The nineteenth-century Respondent Rabbi Jacob Ettlinger therefore makes the distinction between a present and immediate danger on the one hand, and a potential future danger on the other.[4]

Cigarette smoking is harmful, and some rabbinic authorities would accordingly ban it on the religious precept of "Take good heed of yourselves." But a formal ban is not part of rabbinic law, either because the extent of the harmfulness is only now coming to be known, or because the known harmfulness is remote in time. Morphine, for example, is permitted because it gives relief from pain now though it may shorten life later on. On the other hand, use of drugs for other than therapeutic or pain-relieving purposes is harmful to both body and soul. Their addictive properties are physically deleterious; their subversion of sober control of one's actions render them spiritually destructive.

A page from modern Hebrew literature makes vivid a recent historical demonstration of the principle of *pikkuach nefesh*, the religious obligation to protect health. Y. L. Peretz, a novelist of a generation ago, tells the story of how the illustrious Rabbi Israel Salanter acted publicly and dramatically in a situation of crisis in the nineteenth century. Alluding to the Talmud's discussion of the rules for Grace After Meals for three who ate together, Peretz takes the title of that talmudic chapter, "Three Who Ate," as the title of his story as well. He relates the circumstances of the spread of cholera at the time. It's Yom Kippur and the beloved Rabbi Salanter has told his congregation that they must break the fast in order to maintain resistance to the plague. They hesitate; perhaps the plague will pass them by, perhaps they will be strong enough to resist even while fasting. The rabbi saw no alternative. He brought and gave food to the cantor, the sexton and himself. The three ate demonstratively—in order to teach by their unequivocal action what religious law demanded for that time and place.[5]

The point is that the Yom Kippur fast, representative of a fundamental religious discipline least likely to be compromised for any reason, must be set aside for serious health reasons by religious imperative. That the setting aside is itself a mitzvah rather than an evasion thereof is made clear by examples throughout, but poignantly by the following illustration: Eating bread on Passover is another fundamental prohibition in Judaism. Only unleavened bread, *matzah*, may be eaten, and, at the Seder night the obligatory consumption thereof is preceded by the blessing uttered before performing such ritual mitzvot, "Blessed art Thou, Lord our God, Sovereign of the universe, Who hast sanctified us by Thy commandments and commanded us concerning the eating of matzah." Among the stories of religious faith and heroism emerging from the awful Holocaust days is the report of Jewish death-camp inmates who, taking up a morsel of bread on Passover that might keep them alive another day, summoned the strength to recite first "... hast sanctified us by Thy commandments and commanded us concerning preservation of life and health."

· 3 ·

Prayer and Concern for the Ill

Judaism may indeed be a practical, this-worldly religion and a rational system of thought and action, but it gives equal place to the power of prayer. God's healing work through either ordinary Providence or miraculous intercession is as much a reality as the pragmatic, human ministrations.

Like the pithy statement in another mishnaic context, "All is foreseen but freedom is given,"[1] which sets forth the paradox of God's foreknowledge and man's free will, so human efforts at healing and God's ultimate power in the effectiveness or otherwise of this healing are simultaneously affirmed. Our poor ability to comprehend notwithstanding, God is both omnipotent and benevolent, and so we pray that our success be "His will."

There are of course several attempts at comprehending the paradox, at understanding why and when God might bless our efforts and either assure or alter the course of nature. He gives His blessing, whether in response to prayer or without it, when grace is deserved or undeserved.

Taking another look at that essential verse in Exodus (15:26), "If you will hearken to . . . the commandments . . . none of the diseases . . . will I inflict upon you, for I am the Lord thy Healer," it is interesting to hear the Talmud's observation: "But if the diseases are not inflicted, who needs 'the Lord [to be] thy Healer'? The meaning is, if you don't hearken, and I do inflict these diseases, then I am the Lord thy Healer." Then, that is, if you turn in penitence and prayer, I am the Lord your Healer. Or, with slightly less of a supernatural valence, the Midrash (*Mekhilta*) offers: "I am the Lord thy Healer, and I teach you Torah and Commandments which will save you from these diseases—like the physician who says to his patient 'Don't eat this or that, for it might cause this or that disease.'" Similarly, we are taught: "It [obedience] is healing for the body" (Prov. 3:8).[2] In this spirit, prayer helps not by changing the course of nature on behalf of a particular individual, but by bringing the individual in line with divine principles of wholesomeness.

The same naturalist causality is seen in the Talmud's understanding of other apparently supernatural sequences. When the battle against the Amalekites went well for Israel (Ex. 17:11) only "while the hands of Moses were raised," or, when the Israelites were healed of the bite of the fiery serpent "when they gazed at the copper serpent" raised aloft on a banner (Numb. 21:9)—in both cases, says the Talmud (*Rosh HaShanah* 29a): "Do you think it was really the upraised hands of Moses—or the upward gaze to the banner—that saved or healed? No, but when the people look heavenward and subject their hearts to their Father in heaven they are healed." Certainly this is a fundamental teaching, that physical well-being comes from—or comes back again from—subjecting one's heart to God and following the precepts of right living or righteous living.

If, nonetheless, well-being is lost and divine intercession is needed, prayer is resorted to. Then, either God's compassion or the person's merit is evoked to bring about healing. Again, it is no virtue to rely on prayer or miracles alone, for human effort must continue apace. "We may not rely on miracles" is a consistent talmudic teaching, as well as "one should not stand in a dangerous place and say 'a miracle will happen.'" Or, as another passage has it, "I speak to you with reason, and you [instead] tell me 'Heaven will show mercy (and rescue me)!'"[3]

Prayer comes naturally and is taught as a matter of course. The model of brevity was Moses' prayer on Miriam's behalf: "God, please heal her" (Numb. 12:12). Jeremiah prays for healing—"Heal me O Lord and I shall be healed"—and his words, converted into the plural form so that the congregation and its individuals may pray for one another, are prescribed for thrice-daily recital in the Amidah, the Standing Prayer: "Heal us O Lord and we shall be healed." While this is a statutory prayer, prescribed for all to say as a fixed liturgy, it also affords the opportunity of specification, of offering a prayer for a particular individual.

The usual prayer for a particular individual is the *Mi SheBerakh* supplication, recited when the Torah scroll is on the Reader's desk. "May God Who blessed our ancestors Abraham, Isaac and Jacob, Sarah, Rebecca, Rachel and Leah, bless and heal"—and here the individual is mentioned by name. Interestingly, the name by which a man is formally called to the Torah is by first name/son of/father's first name (e.g., David ben Abraham). For the purposes of this prayer one is referred to by first name/son of/mother's first name (David ben Sarah). A reason given for this customary practice is that the mother more than the father is symbolic of compassion; even the word "*rachem*," to have mercy, is popularly associated with "*rechem*," the womb. The prayer asks for *r'fuat ha-nefesh ur'fuat ha-guf*, "healing of the soul and healing of the body"—a significant coupling in terms of the overall theme of this book.

As indicated, the *Mi SheBerakh* prayer is ordinarily recited in the presence of the Torah scroll, which means on Monday and Thursday mornings when the Torah is read in the synagogue. It was originally not done on the Sabbath, when *R'faenu* ("Heal us O Lord") and other prayers of the weekday *Amidah* are also not said, because the Sabbath is a "day of delight" to be relatively free of serious supplications. But a way was found to offer the prayer nonetheless by adding a phrase to the text such as "though Sabbath ought not be a time for crying out." Thus the mood of the day was preserved.

If the Book of Proverbs in the Bible has much to say about prudence and the health of soul and body, the Book of Psalms is an ample source of prayer for God's help in sustaining or retaining health and deliverance. For this reason, "reciting Psalms" became a natural practice in the procedure of prayer by a patient or on his behalf. Particular chapters would be selected or Psalms recited at random, since their overall theme is dependence upon God whether in praise or in supplication. "Saying *Tehillim*," then, became a mode for intercessory prayer, especially by friends or a community on behalf of one of its members.

Remarkable, by the way, is the Talmud's teaching that it is better not to pray for the continued life of one who is in unbearable pain. While no action may ever be taken to shorten life and thus spare the patient pain and suffering, one may pray that God end his life, or cease praying that God keep him in life. This was the example of the humble maid of the dying Rabbi Judah ha-Nasi, which example the Talmud praises.[4]

The Talmud in fact introduces the category of *tefillat shav*, a "futile prayer," wherein one prays for some change in what has already irreversibly happened. Two examples given are: When pregnancy is in its advanced stages, it is wrong to pray that the child be a male, since the sex of the child has already been determined; or, when hearing that there's a house on fire down the block, it's wrong to pray that "it not be my house." To do so would be to ask God to reverse a process, to change the past rather than present or future.

Sympathetic prayer by others has a value in itself, and it is part of a larger sympathetic act, that of *Bikkur Holim*. Visiting the sick is a distinct mitzvah, a mitzvah with palpable social benefit in addition to its religious value. As the talmudic passage made part of the daily prayer service puts it: "These are the commandments, the fruits [dividends] of which are enjoyed in this world, but the principal remains for the next world: Honoring father and mother, doing deeds of kindness . . . giving hospitality to wayfarers, visiting the sick, escorting the dead to their resting place, praying with devotion, making peace between man and his fellow . . ."

The mitzvah even helps us in *imitatio Dei*, since concern for the sick is part of the merciful attributes of God Himself. The Talmud: "'Ye shall walk after the Lord your God' (Deut. 13:5). Can one walk after the Divine Presence? [It means] imitate the qualities of the Holy One, Blessed be He. . . . Just as He visited the sick (e.g., the Lord appeared to Abraham [after his circumcision], Gen. 18:1), so shall you visit the sick . . ."

Elsewhere in the Talmud the mitzvah is underscored in different ways; we are even told that each visitor relieves the patient of a fraction of his illness.[5] It is Nachmanides who specifies that, as an additional purpose of the visit, prayers are recited, and the Code of Jewish Law incorporates this element. But the primary purpose of visiting is to perform an act of kindness (hence, Maimonides locates the source of this mitzvah in "Love thy neighbor as thyself"). The visit shows human concern and enables one to act on this concern in assuring that the patient's medical and personal needs are attended to. In the Abridged Code of Jewish Law, some of the details are spelled out:

"It is a religious duty to visit the sick . . . Even a 'great man' should visit a less important person; even many times a day . . . He who visits frequently is praiseworthy, but not if it troubles the patient . . . The essential feature of this mitzvah is to attend to the patient's needs, to determine what he needs for his benefit, and to give him the pleasure of one's company . . . also to consider his condition and to pray for mercy on his behalf. The visitor should speak with discretion and tact, so as neither to revive him (with false hopes) nor depress him (with words of despair) . . . One should not visit a patient whose condition is an embarrassment to him or for whom conversation is difficult . . . but should call by to make inquiry regarding his condition or his needs . . ."[6]

Though the mitzvah devolves upon every individual (not just the rabbi or chaplain), Jewish communities have, historically, established "societies" for that purpose. The Bikkur Cholim Society of each community would make sure that no patient was neglected and would visit to offer both company and attention to needs.

The mitzvah is not fulfilled by a phone call, it was pointed out in a recent Responsum; although that does have its value, it cannot substitute for a personal presence. Awareness that others care and take the trouble to visit has a salutary effect on the patient's outlook, and his outlook has a salutary effect on his recovery. The human presence and cheering word are part of the therapeutic process—indeed, they "relieve a patient of a fraction of his illness."

· 4 ·

Judaism and Health

Judaism holds medicine and physicians in high esteem. This is a truism, and the reasons for it are manifold.

From biblical times, the *kohanim* (priests) were custodians of public health, wardens in charge of the social-hygiene regulations that feature prominently in Leviticus and elsewhere. And if a health factor is discerned in the dietary laws and rules of sexual relations, then a large proportion of the 613 biblical commandments can be said to be hygienic in intent. These include prevention of epidemics, suppression of venereal diseases, frequent washing, care of the skin, strict sanitary and even quarantine provisions. Contagion was prevented by detailed rules of precautionary or temporary isolation, burning or scalding of infected garments and utensils, and scrupulous inspection and purification of the diseased person after recovery. Even contact with a corpse or carrion required a cleansing period and process. If the hygienic and ritual purity of the Bible do indeed overlap, then health and medicine are very much part of the Jewish tradition.

And since the Talmud is, in the Jewish tradition, both heir to the Bible and the lens through which the Bible is perceived, we find the same health/medicine preoccupation continued there. Talmudic medicine is ample in diagnosis and treatment of diseases, but its major contribution is, like that of the Bible, in the prevention of disease and in the care of community health.

"Bodily cleanliness leads to spiritual cleanliness," says the Talmud more than once (*Avodah Zarah* 20b, TJ *Shabbat* 1:3, 3b), and "The washing of hands and feet in the morning is more effective than any remedy" (*Shabbat* 108b). In order to properly apply biblical law on matters of dietary and hygienic provisions, the rabbis had to become experts on human and animal anatomy and pathology, so that a broad knowledge of these fields is reflected in the Talmud, and many therapeutic regimens are recommended.

35

The Jewish dietary laws—the laws of kosher and nonkosher—belong in our discussion of health and medicine, though the Bible assigns only a spiritual reason for their observance. We are told to "distinguish between the unclean animal and the clean" in order to "be holy for I the Lord your God am holy." The persistent theme among cultural historians has, nonetheless, been that hygienic and sanitary considerations are the motivation for the institution of the dietary laws. They point to the risk of trichinosis from pork products and other diseases from shellfish. The laws against *t'refah*, an animal "torn" by a predatory beast, or *n'velah*, the carcass of an animal that died of itself, seem to have obvious sanitary purposes.

The discussion took an interesting turn in the nineteenth century, as exemplified by the reference in *The Talmud and the Science of Medicine* by Judah Katzenelson.[1] People claim, he writes, that the dietary laws of the Bible show only the great wisdom of Moses, that Moses understood the rules of epidemiology. Aware that disease could be transmitted by an animal that dies of itself or is preyed upon by another, he banned these to the Israelites to keep them physically healthy. This argument, Katzenelson claimed, reckons without the facts of the biblical context. The verse reads: "Thou shalt not eat any *n'velah*; to the alien within thy gates shalt thou give it, that he may eat of it. For a holy nation art thou unto the Lord thy God" (Deut. 14:21). Well, if Moses' intent were to prevent the spread of disease, he would never have permitted it to the "alien within thy gates." Clearly, the purpose is spiritual, to inculcate holiness by this discipline, as the verse itself insists.

The point is sharper when this verse is compared with another: "There shall be one law, for you and for the alien in your midst" (Numb. 15:16). Both were to be equal before the civil law of the Torah, but these dietary provisions were "denominational," something for the Israelites alone.

To return to the Talmud as the font of Jewish tradition in this matter, many of its rabbis were themselves physicians, transmitting the best of medical knowledge available at the time. They sifted the lore; for example, they accepted Greek input but rejected its humoral pathology for an anatomic one. They made room for Persian and Babylonian influence—in terms of amulets, demons and the evil eye—but generally acted on scientific and empirical grounds. A separatist sect at the time were the Essenes, which probably means healers (*"Issi'im,"* from *assa*), who studied and collected herbs and roots for healing purposes, though prayer, mystic formulas and faith were their chief remedies, and their influence is reflected in the New Testament. The Talmud refers to two types of physician, the ordinary *rofei* and the *rofei umman*, the surgeon. Mention is made of *batei shayish*, operating rooms walled with marble for cleanliness, and sleeping drugs (*samma de-shinta*) were used as anesthetics.[2]

The Talmud's appreciation of the physician relates to this skill and usefulness, of course, but much more. "Whoever is in pain, let him go to the physician" (*Bava Kamma* 46b). The physician, in turn, should receive adequate fees, because "A physician who takes nothing is worth nothing" (*ibid.*, 85a). Unless, of course, the patient is needy. The Talmud describes the contemporary Abba Ummana as a reputable physician and a charitable man. So as not to discourage needy patients, he had a box hanging on his outside wall where one could put in, unnoticed, the medical fee he thought he could afford. From poor students Abba Ummana would take no money at all and, if given, would return it to them for use in convalescence (*Ta-'anit* 21b). Perhaps most important as an indication of the doctor's special role, the licensed physician was not liable in Jewish law for damages caused in unintended mistreatment, provided proper care was taken (*Sanhedrin* 84b).

This is related, of course, to the doctor's obligation to heal. What was taken for granted through the generations was made explicit by a rabbinic ruling in the nineteenth century: The communal court could coerce physicians to give free medical service to the poor if they would not do so voluntarily.[3] And the sick themselves and the community at large share in the obligation. The Code of Jewish Law prescribes that the sick may not refuse these free services when required for healing, and that, while use of charitable funds to build a synagogue takes precedence over other purposes, the needs of the indigent sick come before even that.[4]

While the Talmud's authority held firm in matters legal and moral, in medicine it taught principle rather than details. Just as talmudic physicians would not accept uncritically the prevailing remedies, so medieval doctors regarded the diagnoses and prescriptions in the Talmud as based on the knowledge of, and applicable to, that time only. Again in the *Shulhan Arukh*, Rabbi Joseph Caro affirms that the medicines and personal habits of talmudic Babylonia were different from those of medieval European communities.[5] Others before and after him point out that conditions and ways of living "have changed," and that talmudic prescriptions are merely suggestions based on contemporary medical knowledge. The religious imperative is to heal, and for that the best scientific state-of-the-art information must be invoked.

On the other hand, medieval Jewish physicians were not above utilizing methods of healing that were current but not at all scientific. Despite religious opposition to superstitious practices, talmudic authorities of the stature of Rava and Abayei agreed that "nothing done for the purposes of healing is to be forbidden on grounds of superstition" (*Shabbat* 67a). Even biblical prohibitions against magic and sorcery were declared not applicable to the sacred purposes of healing. Amulets and charms and even incantations were tolerated; many bizarre practices of the common folklore were indulged in. Except, says Trachtenberg in his classic study, for the use of blood as a remedy in internal medicine: Because of religious strictures, human or animal blood was never ingested as a remedy, all the more ironic in view of recurrent blood libels.[6] But the physician's relentless search for *r'fuah b'dukah um'nusah*, the scientific-empirical relief of pain and symptomatology, pushed back the frontiers and led to the advances of modern medicine.

Aside from obvious usefulness, doctors enjoy a special reverence in the Judaic scheme of things because they figure in halakhic determinations. Since the Yom Kippur fast is set aside on the word of the physician, even when the patient feels he is strong enough to fast, the physician becomes a halakhic factor. Seeing that a threat to life or health sets aside all ritual provisions, the physician is crucial to these halakhic decisions. This gives him a preeminence in Jewish tradition to match his prominence in Jewish history.

At a conference in Rome under the auspices of the Vatican, I had just finished offering my version of Jewish teaching on the question of abortion. I had touched upon the matter of a life-threatening pregnancy and the warrant for abortion under those circumstances. A Catholic woman physician at the conference rose to challenge my position. She told of a difficult pregnancy she herself had experienced: The doctor had counseled abortion but her priest forbade it. She listened to her priest, and the story had a happy ending; the child was born without incident. I was nonplussed, not being able to respond theoretically to her personal experience. But there was a Catholic priest who also rose to his feet to come to my defense. He said to her, "As a Catholic woman, you are duty-bound to listen to your priest, who will tell you that an abortion is wrong. But a Jewish woman is equally duty-bound to listen to her rabbi, who will tell her that Jewish law forbids her to put her life in danger; that it requires her to obey the doctor in this matter, even if the doctor later turns out to have been mistaken." I remain indebted to that anonymous priest who was so well versed on this point. He saved the day for me and clarified the role the physician occupies in the Jewish scheme of things.

There are, of course, limitations to our reliance upon the good doctor. These are interesting in themselves, because it means we "listen to the doctor" only when the doctor is more "lenient" than the religious law. For example, as said above, if the doctor is too strict with regard to Yom Kippur, saying that the patient is well enough to fast and the patient doesn't think so, we dismiss the doctor's advice and stay on the safe side. We give the patient the benefit of the doubt and tell him not to fast. Similarly, the laws of circumcision reflect this difference. Circumcision of an infant is designated for the eighth day after birth, even if that day is a Sabbath or Yom Kippur. But a slight degree of jaundice makes the operation a hazardous one, so the *b'rit* is postponed until it's safe to have it. Now, if the doctor declares it safe to proceed with the circumcision, but the officiating Mohel, using criteria of Jewish law which are stricter—that is, more lenient in that the postponement is allowed—insists that the baby has not yet reached the safe level, then we reject the doctor's assessment and stay on the safe side.

It must, incidentally, be added that the Mohel's performance of the circumcision itself is preferred to the doctor's for medical as well as religious reasons. Opponents of the routine practice of infant circumcision point to an incidence, though statistically very small, of mishaps. This does not apply to the work of the Mohel who is, of course, necessary for the ritual dimension, but who combines high surgical standards with specialized experience.[7]

The more serious limitation on the doctor concerns the thrust of his role. Since he has "permission" and thus the "obligation" to heal, his role is that of healer only. This means he has a mandate to heal, not to cooperate in what is actually suicide or homicide—hastening death because of the wishes of patient or family. Neither may he despair prematurely—as in the story told by Rabbi Eisel Harif, a famous scholar in nineteenth-century Poland who was attended by an eminent physician. At a certain point, the physician pronounced the situation hopeless and withdrew from the case. Notwithstanding the doctor's grave prognosis, R. Eisel recovered completely. When their paths crossed again, R. Eisel said of him, "This is no doctor. He does not treat patients; he abandons them."

Rabbi Moses Sofer (d. 1839) once expressed himself with regard to the medical profession in a way that accounts for both the readiness to heed the doctor's admonitions and to disregard his despair or deny him infallibility. Doctors, he said, may know medicine well but don't know the patient. Since medicine is more of an art than a skill, success lies in knowing the variables.

If the doctor is to be relied upon so implicitly, it follows, too, that one ought to seek the best, or better, doctor. One Responsum, from early in this century, illustrates the point. A woman had a narrow cervical os and required Caesarian section for parturition. She and her husband had inquired of the rabbi whether they could use contraceptive devices in order to space the births, since having a Caesarian every year or so would be hazardous. The rabbi wasn't sure of how to answer, so he consulted with a greater rabbi in the larger city. Meanwhile, the couple did not wait for his reply, and another pregnancy occurred. This time a normal delivery was possible. When they communicated this to the rabbi, he scolded them for having listened to their local doctor in the first place. Just as he had consulted the more learned rabbi, they too should have referred their medical question to the "professor," i.e., to the specialist in the big city![8]

Seeking the best in medical care, even obtaining a "second opinion," thus becomes part of the religious imperative. An organization was recently formed in Israel called "Medicine in Accordance with Jewish Law," which bridges the ancient and the modern worlds. It gathers data in computerized records on the skill and effectiveness record of physicians in various specialties.[9] Instituted by and for its ultraorthodox clients, it concerns itself with expected matters such as autopsy and abortion, but—in keeping with this perception of religious obligation—it also enables them to seek and find the very best in medical care.

· 5 ·

Jews and Medicine

The large variety of climates, environments and customs to which Jews were exposed in their migrations in exile enhanced the development of their medical knowledge and experience. The prevalence, for example, of eye diseases in the Orient greatly encouraged the development of ophthalmology, which the Jews then brought with them to Europe.

The contribution of Jewish doctors in the medieval period lay not only in their individual achievements, but in their work as translators and transmitters of Greek medicine to Europe. Jewish physicians were proficient in Greek, Latin, Arabic and Hebrew, which enabled them to translate most of the Arab and Greek medical works into Hebrew and Latin and vice versa. The English scholar Roger Bacon (d. 1292) declared that Christian physicians were ignorant in comparison with Jewish colleagues because they lacked knowledge of Hebrew and Arabic. Mosellanus, in his rectorial address at the University of Leipzig in 1518, urged Christian medical students to learn Hebrew so that they might study the medical lore "hidden in the libraries of the Jews." Aside from linguistic cosmopolitanism, the close religious and family ties linking the various Jewish communities helped spread medical knowledge. As merchants and travelers, the Jews met the best minds of the time and acquainted themselves with drugs, plants and remedies from around the world.[1]

Though Jewish physicians suffered from persecution and restriction, they were held in high esteem by their non-Jewish colleagues. Countless regulations, papal bulls and royal ordinances forbade Jewish physicians to practice among non-Jews, to hold official positions and, later, to study at universities. Nonetheless, they continued to excel in their profession and attained high positions at the courts of the very authorities who preached against them.

The large numbers of Jewish physicians during these centuries is due to

41

the fact that the profession was regarded as a spiritual vocation compatible with the career of rabbi. Rabbinic scholars, who felt it improper to earn a living from religious teaching, took up medicine as an honorable means of employment.

The curriculum of talmudic schools often included the philosophies and sciences of the day. The Babylonian Talmud centers of Sura and Pumbeditha flourished in the Byzantine era, and Greek medicine was a staple item. Asaph HaRofe, who lived in the Middle East in the sixth century, was among the more famous physicians. He founded a medical school and authored a work—the oldest known medical book in Hebrew—which offered all the then known Greek, Babylonian, Egyptian and Persian medicine of the pre-Arabic period. One of the most outstanding medical personalities after the Arabic conquest was Isaac Israeli, whose works were brought to Europe and remained classics for several hundred years. Uninfluenced by the Arab culture was the medical study center that flourished in Salerno, southern Italy, from the ninth to the twelfth century, where Shabbetai Donnolo's famous work, *Sefer HaYakar*, lists 120 different remedies and their composition. The "Golden Age" of Jewry in Spain (eighth to fifteenth centuries) witnessed the elevation of Jews to high positions in Moorish and Christian courts. They served as physicians to the sultans and caliphs, as well as statesmen, philosophers and poets. Of the latter, Judah HaLevi (eleventh century) exerted great influence as a physician, poet and philosopher.

The most important Jewish physician of the period was, of course, Moses Maimonides. We have already met him as a philosopher and a legal codifier, where his influence is greatest. In 1170 he became personal physician to the family of Sultan Saladin of Egypt and continued to serve them until his death in 1204. Though his philosophy and, much more so, his legal-religious works are what earned him his continuing eminence in Jewish thought, he wrote ten medical works as well. His professions dovetail, because his concept of medicine is based on the conviction that a healthy soul requires a healthy body. One's intellectual and moral capabilities can then be developed toward greater knowledge of God and the ethical life. Healing, to Maimonides, is the art of repairing both the defects of the body and the turmoil of the mind. The physician therefore should have both technical knowledge and the skill and intuition to understand the patient's personality and life-style. Though leaning heavily on the medicine of the ancient Greeks, he warns against blind acceptance of authorities and calls for clear thought and experimentation.

Both Isaac Israeli and Maimonides, for whom the Talmud was the unquestioned authority, were independent in their quest for medical knowledge, as indicated above. Galen was revered in the field, and scholars warned against uncritical use of talmudic remedies because they are not equally effective in all places and times. More important, they are not binding as are religious precepts, since they are based on ever-developing technical know-how.

Jewish centers of learning were established in southern France in the twelfth and thirteenth centuries—Avignon, Lunel, Montpellier, Beziers. Papal bulls and synod decrees alternated in forbidding and then allowing Jewish physicians to practice. Again, the principal service rendered was the translation of Arabic works into Hebrew and Latin, such as the Canon of Avicenna of the eleventh century, but translation was accompanied by great scholarly activity. The medical school of Montpellier was founded largely by Jewish scholars, portraits of some of whom were included in the marble plaques at the university. Jean Astruc (d. 1766), professor of medicine there and later physician to Louis XV, and the Saporta and Sanchez families, for many generations on the faculty there until their emigration to the French colonies of America, were among the prominent names. Also, Jewish women physicians attained fame during this time—Sarah La Migresse in Paris, thirteenth century; Sarah de Saint Gilles in Marseilles, fourteenth century; and Sarah of Wuerzburg and Rebekah Zerlin of Frankfort, both fifteenth century.

Back in Spain, the list of prominent physicians is long indeed. Nathan ben Joel Falaquera (thirteenth century) and Abraham ben David Caslari (fourteenth century) wrote important texts, as did Meir Aldabi, another rabbi-philosopher in Toledo. The Marranos and their descendants were leaders and pioneers in medicine in Europe and Asia for several centuries. The sixteenth century was a time of great discovery and progress, and many Jewish refugees from Spain won world-wide reputations elsewhere. Amatus Lusitanus wrote *Centuria*, a description of 700 cases of disease, and fought against superstition and quackery. Many families distinguished themselves: Abraham Zacuto was a famous physician and astronomer, and his grandson Zacutus Lusitanu wrote a seventeen-volume history of medicine as well as a code of ethics for physicians. Dionysus Bundus (d. 1540) fled from Portugal to Antwerp, where he wrote on phlebotomy, while his son Manuel published widely read works on febrile diseases. Then there was Luis Mercado, who wrote *De Veritate* in 1604, a medico-philosophic opus, and Isaac Cardozo, court physician to Philip IV in Madrid in the seventeenth century. Also, Francisco Lopez, who wrote on syphilis and bubonic plague, and Roderigo Lopez, who became physician to Elizabeth of England. Roderigo de Castro (1627) wrote on gynecology and was physician to the king of Denmark. His son Benedict became physician to the queen of Sweden. Orobio de Castro was a famous physician in Amsterdam, while Jacob de Castro (d. 1762), who became a fellow of the Royal Society of England, wrote on the therapeutic qualities of quinine. Jacob Pereira was a pioneer in the education of deaf-mutes, to the improvement of whose plight he devoted his life. Another Marrano traveled as far as Russia: Antonio Sanchez became physician to Catherine II in 1740. Others went to Turkey (the Hamon family), East India (Garcia de Orta, Cristoval d'Acosta) and Italy.

In Italy, several of the Jewish physicians were also rabbis and community leaders, especially in Rome, Ferrara, Mantua and Genoa. At a time when most other European universities were closed to Jews, those of Padua and Perugia were open to them. They served as personal physicians to popes, cardinals, bishops and dukes. Here too the periods of leniency were followed by periods of restriction and harassment, but the Jews earned the reputation for unselfish devotion to their calling, especially during times of epidemic. To mention a few of the Italian Jewish physicians of the fifteenth–sixteenth centuries: Saladino d'Acosta was a leading pharmacologist, whose book was the basic text until the eighteenth century. Bonet de Lattes (d. 1515) was physician to Popes Alexander VI and Leo X, while serving as rabbi to the Jewish community of Rome. David de Pomis (d. 1593) was physician to Pope Pius IV; Eliagus Montalto (d. 1616) was the same for Grand Duke Ferdinand of Florence and later to Queen Marie de Medici of France. He wrote *Archipathologia* on nervous and mental disorders. Roderigo de Fonseca diagnosed internal diseases; Benjamin Mussafia was physician to the Danish King Christian IV and was a distinguished rabbi. Rabbi Jacob Zahalon of Ferrara wrote *Otzar HaHayyim* describing disease and redefining the moral obligations of doctors. Joseph Delmedigo, a pupil of Galileo, became physician to Prince Radziwil of Poland, while the family Conegliano were prominent in Venice in the eighteenth century.

Up north, the grand duke of Brandenburg permitted Jews to enter the University of Frankfort am Oder in the seventeenth century. The most famous alumnus was Tobias ben Moses Cohn, who took his degree in Padua. He was physician to five successive sultans in Constantinople, and bequeathed us his *Ma'aseh Tuvia*, an encyclopedic work on medicine and science. Marcus Eliezer Bloch was a famous general practitioner in Berlin in the eighteenth century, as was Gumperz Levison in England and

Sweden, Elias Henschel, a pioneer in modern obstetrics, and Marcus Herz, an outstanding philosopher.

The gates of European medical schools were thrown open to the Jews in 1782 when Joseph II of Austria proclaimed the Act of Tolerance and when the French Revolution brought emancipation. Jewish doctors then made enormous contributions to medical advancement. Though classroom doors were opened, many portals to academic recognition were still closed, as were "establishment" specialties. As a result, Jews cultivated less popular fields, such as dermatology and venereology, and later biochemistry, immunology, psychiatry and "microscopy"—that is, hematology, histology and microscopic pathology. The illustrious names then included Ludwig Traube in experimental pathology, Robert Remak in embryology, Moritz Romberg in neuropathology, Benedict Shelling, Auerbach, Edinger and Oppenheim in neurology. Jacob Henle described the germ theory of infection, Gabriel Valentin enriched every branch of basic science, Julius Colinheim traced pus cells to the blood; Kronecker, Heidenheim, Zuntz and Munk were trailblazers in physiology, as was Carl Weigert in bacteriology. Ferdinand Widal devised a test for the prevention of typhoid fever; Mordecai Haffkine, vaccines against cholera and plague; and Wasserman and Ehrlich, antitoxins and immunology.

Jews were prominent in clinical medicine as well: Bamberger in cardiology, Hermann Senator in kidney diseases, Rosenbach in functional disease; Edward Henoch in pediatrics, Boginsky in nutrition, Max Kassowitz in congenital syphilis and rickets. Adam Politzer founded the specialty of otolaryngology, and George Gerson and Karl Koller excelled in ophthalmology. Kristeller, Wilhelm Freund and Leopold Landau excelled in obstetrics-gynecology, and Leopold Freund founded X-ray therapy in 1897. Wolfeer, James Israel and Leopold van Dittel devised new surgical techniques and instruments.

In France, Julius Sichel established the first eye clinic in Paris in 1830; Michael Levy pioneered in public health and George Hayen in hematology. In Denmark, there was Jacobson in anatomy, Hannover in occupational diseases, Salomonsen and Hirschprung in pediatrics. In Holland, it was Van Deen in physiology; in Italy, Lambroso in anatomy; Hirszfeld in the same field in Poland, with Goldflam in neurology and Zamenhof in ophthalmology. In America, the Jewish contribution to medicine in the nineteenth century was modest, but it was discernible in the organization and the founding of hospitals. Isaac Hays (d. 1879) was one of the founders of the AMA. Jacob de Silva Solis-Cohen was the father of laryngology, and

Abraham Jacobi was the founder of the American Pediatric Society, then president of the AMA.

The early twentieth century saw Wasserman and Ehrlich being joined by Cassimir Funk, the father of "vitamins," and Joseph Goldberger, who introduced nicotinic acid for pellagra, as well as Alfred Hess with Vitamin C for scurvy and Gustav Bucky, who invented the X-ray diaphragm that bears his name. The first Jewish doctors in the U.S. were of Sephardic origin; then came the immigrants from Germany in the late nineteenth century, followed by those from Russia after the pogroms of the 1880s.

The majority of those who escaped Nazi Germany in the 1930s and 40s came to the United States or Israel. This was the golden age of scientific medicine, with antibiotics and cortisone and advances in molecular biology and medical technology. The U.S. welcomed the newcomers. Jewish hospitals—Mt. Sinai in New York, Mt. Sinai and Michael Reese in Chicago —as well as non-Jewish hospitals and research centers and universities absorbed them. By the mid-sixties, Jewish doctors constituted about nine percent of the physician population in the United States, well over three times their percentage in the general population.

Hospital affiliation has a history of its own, documented by a contemporary scholar.[2] Medieval Jewish communities had hospitals similar to those of Christian societies, namely inns to house poor or sick travelers and to nurse the ailing poor of the community itself; others were treated at home. The first hospitals built exclusively for the sick under Jewish auspices arose in the late eighteenth century in European countries of the Enlightenment, where conditions of life were relatively stable. There were such Jewish hospitals in most countries of Europe by 1933, with the pattern continuing in North America. Here the rationale differed: The original motivation for the establishment of Jewish hospitals was to provide a compatible environment for Jewish patients, in keeping with their specific needs. With the greater degree of assimilation in America, this ethnic or religious need diminished; the justification for special involvement in building and maintaining hospitals was then to provide professional opportunities for Jewish physicians who suffered discrimination at existing institutions. When such discrimination was far less of a problem after 1950, the rationale shifted again. Jewish sponsorship of a hospital is now primarily a Jewish service to society.

The Jewish contribution to American medicine is the subject of many volumes and of a long entry in the *Encyclopedia Judaica*. Like the sketch of Jewish involvement in world medical history relayed above, their contributions locally are detailed in entries there, covering all fields of medicine.[3] These are, notably, chemical immunology (penicillin, streptomycin, neomycin), wherein Bela Schick, Jonas Salk and Albert Sabin conquered diphtheria and polio; hematology (discoveries of blood groups)—Landsteiner; enabling of transfusions—Witebsky; work on leukemia—Dameshek; cancer—Schwartz; bone marrow transplants—Epstein; hemoglobin—Jaffe; and enzyme deficiencies—Beutler. Also: metabolism and endocrinology (diabetes)—Minkowski; insulin—Barron and Rachmiel Levine; endocrine disturbances—Snapper and Reichlin. Also, heart, lung and kidney diseases, gastroenterology, neurology, dermatology, pediatrics, surgery, ob-gyn, radiology and pathology, as well as public health and education. Such contributions were offered especially in the United States, but also in Canada, England, France, Sweden, Latin America, South Africa and Israel.

Major contributions to the theory and practice of medicine in all its individual and communal aspects continue to be made by modern heirs to Jewish tradition and Jewish history.

· 6 ·

Mental as well as Physical Health

In view of the palpable interaction between *psyche* and *soma*, it is no surprise that mental health is equal to physical health as a halakhic concern. Whatever may be done—say, a violation of the Sabbath—to attend to a health threat may be done as readily for a mental-health hazard. Of course, the danger spoken of must be of a fundamental, not an ordinary or transitory, nature.

The principle is enunciated in the Talmud (*Yoma* 82): *Teiruf da'at*, a threat to mental equilibrium, is to be treated like *pikkuach nefesh*, a threat to one's physical life. The authoritative Nahmanides (thirteenth century) makes this unequivocal: Just as measures in violation of ritual law may be taken for one, they may be taken for the other.[1] In the late seventeenth century, a Responsum gives this principle interesting application. A certain nonkosher soup was reputed to have therapeutic properties; one person insisted he would go out of his mind unless he had some. Rabbi Israel Meir Mizrachi, noting that serious danger to mental health is tantamount to a risk to one's physical well-being, issued a permissive ruling. Let him have the forbidden soup and save his sanity![2]

Other authorities ruled similarly—even in matters of abortion and contraception. In 1913 Rabbi Mordecai Winkler was asked this question and, among other arguments, replied: "Mental-health risk has been definitely equated to physical-health risk (in Jewish law). This woman, who is in danger of losing her mental health unless the pregnancy is interrupted, would accordingly qualify."[3] And using contraceptive devices to prevent a pregnancy that could create serious mental-health risks is approved consistently by the rabbinic authorities.[4]

The contributory role of mental or emotional equilibrium in dealing with physical threats is also acknowledged. The Talmud (*Shabbat* 128b) permits deeds in violation of the Sabbath intended only to calm the psychic concerns of a woman in labor; even unnecessary lights may be kindled, for example, to "set her mind at ease." This is evidenced also by the ruling and accepted practice that the husband, too, must violate the Sabbath to assist his wife. If giving birth is imminent, not only may she violate the ban on Sabbath travel or other activity, but her husband must join her in so doing in order to be present for reassurance and emotional assistance. Further, a physician may break the Sabbath to treat a patient even where other physicians are available, if the patient has confidence only in this particular doctor. The confidence factor is part of the patient's mental state and, though merely subjective, plays a part in his objective physical restoration.

This is related to the larger subject of the "will to live." The patient's state of mind is all important, and even the death-bed confessional reflects that understanding. The confessional is not couched in the declarative but in the conditional mood, since any statement that "I am about to die" weakens the resolve to live and thus shortens the life even by a moment. Rather, the moribund patient says something like "Heal me; but, if not, I prepare myself, etc." For similar reasons, signing a Living Will is classified among actions that may neutralize the psychological factor. Aside from legal and moral problems in signing such documents, there is also some resigning of the will to recover or remain alive.

In the theoretical realm of religious concepts, even sin is an imbalance of the mental state. How could one sin if he were really in command of all his faculties? The Talmud (*Sotah* 3a) says: "A person sins only if seized by a spirit of foolishness." The word here for foolishness (*ru'ach shtut*) is the same word as for lunacy or mental aberration.

Psychotherapy then would seem to be a religio-moral corrective to bring a person back to spiritual as well as mental wholeness. As a field of specialization, psychotherapy has attracted Jewish professional interest to a great degree. On the other hand, traditional religion has looked askance at psychotherapy and its principles, primarily because of the attitudes associated with Sigmund Freud and his school of thought. This kind of conflict can be seen on a "secular" level as well, when the value-system of a therapist is different from that of his patient. Should "therapeutic adultery" be recommended in marriage therapy, for example, when this clashes with the patient's moral system? The disparity between the values of patient and therapist is at times an obstacle to healing, but the wholeness that is sought for the patient should be sought on his terms. Accordingly, an increasing number of religiously committed therapists have entered the field to offer psychotherapy in keeping with the world-view of their subjects. Alternatively, the therapist takes a "nonjudgmental" stance and allows the patient to work out his conflicts or neuroses without having to accept the therapist's assumptions.[5]

Almost by definition, religion teaches conscience and therefore the reality of guilt. But guilt, or too much conscience, causes neuroses, complexes and maladjustments. A distinction must be made between pathological guilt, which needs to be dissipated, and normal guilt, necessary for the health of both individual and society. Pathological guilt does not arise merely from awareness of misdeed, and it is disproportionate to any reality. Normal guilt does arise proportionately from misdeed; though painful, it keeps one from lapsing further and serves as a stimulus to self-improvement.

Thus, healthy guilt feelings and fundamental value systems must be respected; mental health cannot be purchased by eliminating them. But on the principle of *pikkuach nefesh*, other mitzvot are set aside. Observance of the commandment to "honor one's father and mother," for example, can obstruct the progress of family therapy. A child with problems in parental relationships needs to express his deepest feelings to the therapist, sometimes in the presence of the parents. If he suppresses these feelings in keeping with the commandment, therapy cannot proceed. Of course, the halakhic definition of the commandment distinguishes between aggressive disobedience and respectful self-assertiveness. But legitimizing the child's feelings and facilitating their expression is standard therapeutic practice that helps bring about healthier human relations and even a strengthening of the family unit.

The reality of the mental factor is acknowledged in another way. Halakhah considers a person morally culpable only if he is free to act without compulsion. This means that homosexual activity, for example, is a moral offense when freely chosen. If, however, the condition is a result of "sickness" —which very idea is rejected by gay society and by the American Psychiatric Association— then there is no moral blame attached. The prohibition remains firm against homosexual indulgence as a freely chosen act or lifestyle.

Not unrelated to the subject of this chapter is the attitude to the disabled and their treatment in Jewish law and life. Three categories are bracketed together in mishnaic and talmudic law in connection with legal restrictions or exemptions. They are *heresh, shoteh, v'katan*, the deaf-mute, the lunatic and the minor. The minor's restrictions from privilege or exemptions from responsibility are easily remediable. When a male attains the age of majority at thirteen with his bar mitzvah, or a female at age twelve with her bat mitzvah, the disabilities of minor status disappear. Those of a lunatic or imbecile continue, presumably, if the condition is chronic. But there has been much refinement of the law with regard to the first category, the deaf-mute, and this is paradigmatic for other conditions of impairment as well.

First, the Talmud establishes that the *heresh* of the mishnaic law refers to the deaf-mute only, not to one who is either deaf or mute. The rationale of the law to begin with is that one who was born deaf-mute was not able to communicate or be communicated with, hence does not have the requisite knowledge with which to effect documents of contract, of marriage and divorce, or to perform certain ritual acts. If he could either speak or hear, he could overcome these limitations and acquire the knowledge. In subsequent Jewish law, a debate took shape concerning the deaf-mute who was trained to read lips or sign language.

Does this training lift him from the restrictions or exemptions? Some rabbinic authorities preserved the categories of talmudic legislation and ruled that training in lip reading or sign language does not alter his status. Others understood the categories as functional rather than arbitrary and emphatically welcomed the retrained disabled to the ranks of "normal in all matters" like the rest of us.[6] In the family of the famous rabbinic leaders, that of Hatam Sofer, one had taken a stricter position against removing the legal restrictions upon a deaf-mute, though now trained to read lips, while the other begged to differ. Having witnessed firsthand the marvelous facilities and results of modern schools for the purpose, he ruled in favor of declassifying the trainees from the disabled status.[7]

But even for the deaf-mute who had not overcome his inability to communicate, and thus remained in the talmudic category according to all, the provisions of both law and ethics protected his welfare. To begin with, there was the biblical prohibition in Leviticus 19:14: "Thou shalt not curse the deaf." To the rabbinic exegetes this could not have been meant to be taken literally. Who would be so cruel? It must mean something like "Don't curse or slander one who cannot hear to defend himself." Like the second half of the verse, "nor place a stumbling block before the blind," which must mean something like "Don't lead the unwary astray with bad-faith advice," or "Don't tempt with wine one who has taken the Nazirite vow against drinking wine." Other interpreters have understood "*lo t'kallel*, thou shalt not curse" on the basis of the root meaning of the verb, which is *kal*, light. That is, don't take lightly the plight of the deaf or, by extension, the disabled of one kind or another. The verse in Proverbs (17:5) referring to *lo-eg la-rash*, "disdaining the unfortunate," was applied to the ethical infraction of mistreating the afflicted by showing superiority in their presence. One is enjoined, in fact, against walking quickly alongside a crippled person.

The ethical thrust took on an interesting form with respect to some of the legal disabilities of, for example, the deaf-mute. According to talmudic law, the deaf-mute, never having learned to communicate properly, is legally barred from making contracts, from the formal sale or purchase of land, or from contracting marriage or divorce. The latter is a contractual arrangement no less than a romantic one, with promises undertaken and exchanged. Viewing this situation with compassion, the rabbis instituted a "rabbinic marriage contract" on behalf of the handicapped. Constituting themselves as guarantors of the promises that bride and groom would exchange, and calling themselves *avuhon-shel hareshim*, the "fathers of the deaf-mute," they paternalistically took upon themselves the fulfillment of these practical obligations, so that the couple might enjoy a marital relationship even without the biblically stipulated contractual terms.[8]

In more prosaic ways, the law was applied with sympathy for the disabled in ritual matters. If the use of electricity on the Sabbath, or mechanical amplification of sound through microphone, is legally problematic for others, the use of an electric hearing aid for the hard-of-hearing comes under the category of a necessity.[9] It is both life-enhancing and life-saving. The person can protect himself better as he crosses the street, accidents usually occurring where the pedestrian sees all but cannot hear what is approaching unseen. These insights of the law, as well as practical efforts to increase access to buildings and heighten public cooperation on behalf of the handicapped, are embodied in current activities of, for example, the Medical Ethics Committee of New York's Federation of Jewish Philanthropies.

· 7 ·

Marriage and Marital Relations

That the health of body and soul is intertwined is seen most clearly in Jewish attitudes to marriage and sex. Here a fine blending of the physical and spiritual inform the legal and moral precepts, and do so often in opposition to prevailing attitudes.

The Jewish and Christian traditions parted on these matters. Dr. Derrick S. Bailey, an Anglican minister, details the story in his acclaimed book *Sexual Relations in Christian Thought*, where he traces the divergence to the time of St. Paul.[1] Though St. Paul's preachments were directed to the Endtime, he espoused ideas of purity aimed at negating the hedonism and the crass sexual immorality he encountered among the Greeks. His response and prescription went too far in the other direction, and he embraced a dualism uncharacteristic of his Judaic heritage. Dr. Bailey surveys the history and asks rhetorically, "How have we Christians departed so from our Hebraic roots"—and gone so far as to teach that celibacy and virginity are preferable to marriage? Only, he answered, because St. Paul had introduced a dualism into the new faith, whereby emphasis on the body implied a de-emphasis on the soul, and vice versa. If one would be holy, then he must suppress the bodily desires; if he indulges the body he cannot expect to be among the holy.

Add to this the Augustinian elaboration, associating sex with original sin and viewing marriage as relief from concupiscence, and classic Christianity was confirmed as a dualistic system with body and soul at odds with each other.

These attitudes, formulated in basic dogmas were also reflected in practical teachings. If, for example, a woman had been told by her physician that another pregnancy would be hazardous to her health, she would hear her priest counsel abstinence as the best way to avoid such hazard. Since sex remains evil, and it is procreation of children that justifies temporary indulgence in this evil, contraception is unthinkable. Abstinence is the holier course generally, so abstinence is the proper solution to her medical problem.

Rabbinic Responsa for the past two millennia on the subjects of contraception, abortion and marital relations are distilled in the present author's book *Birth Control in Jewish Law*. These collated Responsa yield a comprehensive and consistent view of Jewish attitudes to sex and marriage. A distinct value system emerges as the factors and priorities are weighed by the respondent—say, a composite rabbi representing the historic response to this hypothetical woman. She addresses the rabbi with the question: The doctor claims a pregnancy would be a threat to my life or health. What shall I do?

The rabbi weighs the factors involved. On the one hand, he muses, there's the mitzvah of *p'ru ur'vu*, of "be fruitful and multiply." It's a fundamental imperative. Technically, the imperative falls on the man to fulfill; it is his responsibility. The woman participates in the mitzvah, but she has no legal responsibility to seek opportunities for fulfillment. On the polygamous assumption, Rachel could say to Jacob, "go and fulfill the mitzvah with Leah." Even in monogamous situations, the husband is the one who has to "worry about" it. Alternatively, as discussed elsewhere, the woman's innate maternal desire does not need additional legislation. In either case, the rabbi soon concludes that one side of the scale is weighed down with a strong positive, the mitzvah or desire to procreate.

On the other side of the scale is the negative, the danger to the woman's health in realizing this mitzvah/desire. The couple may not fulfill a mitzvah at the expense of her health, as we have seen in the discussion above. The scale is now balanced: The mitzvah of procreation is canceled by the equally important mitzvah of protection of health; an impasse is reached. Our composite rabbi is momentarily stymied; what should be done? The obvious solution is—abstinence.

But no sooner does that solution suggest itself than it must be rejected out of hand: Abstinence in the Jewish view is a sin. Here the contrast between the Jewish approach and the classic Christian one is sharply apparent. Abstinence is a sin because it is a total suppression of the physical in the name of the spiritual—an unacceptable dualism.

Whence does the rabbi take his view that abstinence is not the proper solution? From awareness of another mitzvah, one that must be added to the first side of the scale and tip it accordingly. This is the mitzvah of marital sex, of *onah*. Sex in marriage is a mitzvah in and of itself, independent of the imperative of *p'ru ur'vu.* This is the mitzvah of conjugal rights, owed by a husband to his wife; it must be placed on the scale alongside the pro-creational duty. The source is Exodus 21:10, where we are told that if a man takes a wife, he must provide her with three goods in return for her having become his wife. He must provide her with food, shelter and con-jugal rights. The conjugal rights are of a given frequency, whether or not procreation is now or ever possible, even when the wife is temporarily or permanently barren.

And, lest the husband feel he can absolve himself with a token fulfill-ment of this pledge, the Mishnah sets forth a recommended frequency, based on the husband's age, health and occupation. If he now wants to change his occupation from what it was before marriage—from one that allowed him to remain home more to one which requires him to be away from home more often—the Talmud says he may not make this occupa-tional change without his wife's permission.[2] With the mitzvah of marital sex involved, he cannot make a unilateral decision in this matter. In the Middle Ages, when asceticism—as opposed to abstinence—became popular among Christians, many Jews wanted to do likewise. They would deny themselves food, drink and sex in the name of asceticism, self-denial being good for the soul. Into this question the rabbis entered and said, in effect, if you want to deny yourselves food and drink, that's your decision. But sex? That's not up to you. It "takes two to tango," and you can't be "virtuous" at your wife's expense. With these and similar talmudic provisions in mind, the responding rabbi knew he could not counsel abstinence.

He could not, moreover, because of a ruling such as this: What if a woman, experiencing difficulty in finding a marriage partner, wants to make a deal with a particular man? What if she says to him, in effect: "I know that if you marry me the Torah requires you to provide me with food, shelter and sex. But I don't need food and shelter from you. I have my own career, my own source of support. Just marry me and I will forgo the first or second of those obligations." In the case of such a prenuptial stipulation, the Talmud says: The marriage is valid and the stipulation is valid. But what if she specifies the contrary: "I know the Torah requires you to pro-vide me with food, shelter and conjugal rights. But I'm mostly interested in a means of support. Marry me, give me the food and shelter, and I'll do without the sex." In this case, says the Talmud, the marriage is valid but the agreement is null and void! We pay no attention to a stipulation such as this, because it amounts to contracting an abstinent marriage.[3] An ab-stinent marriage is a contradiction in terms, and to contract such a mar-riage is to make a "stipulation against the Torah." The Torah's concept of marriage is a physical-spiritual one. It is a spiritual relationship on a physical foundation.

And so this mitzvah of ongoing conjugal rights joins with the procreational imperative to heavily weigh down the scale. The impasse remains: How fulfill these objectives and yet avoid hazard?

The rabbi now abandons any suggestion of abstinence. What then? Perhaps, it occurs to him, contraception? He no sooner contemplates this solution than he confronts a formidable set of objections. Contraception implies onanism, and onanism is condemned in the Bible, more so in the Talmud, and even more so in the Zohar, the mystic tradition.

The word "onanism" was coined as a result of theological and literary references in Christianity to the act of Onan described in Genesis 38. There we are told of Er and Onan, sons of Judah, and of how Tamar, the childless widow of Er, was given to Onan so that offspring might be born in the name of his late brother. But Onan, declining to fulfill this "levirate" duty, "when he went to his brother's wife, would spill [it] on the ground, lest he should give seed for his brother. And the thing which he did was evil in the sight of the Lord, and He slew him also" (Gen. 38:9, 10).

The passage served as the basis for censure of several related evils in Christian Church doctrine. In the fourth century, Epiphanius, bishop in Cyprus, invoked the story of that "immense and frightful crime" of Onan; and St. Jerome writes that Onan "did a detestable thing." But it was the influential St. Augustine who applied the passage to contraception in marriage by any means: It is lawless and shameful to lie with one's wife where the conception of offspring is avoided; "this is what Onan, son of Judah, did, and God slew him for it." From then on, Catholic moralists in various times and places condemned either contraception or coitus interruptus as the sin of onanism. These culminated in the citation by Pope Pius XI in *Casti Connubii* (1930), his all-important encyclical on marital conduct, where he affirms: "Holy Writ itself testifies that the Divine Majesty pursued this wicked crime with detestation and punished it with death, as St. Augustine recalls." Within the Protestant tradition, it was primarily Calvin who adverted to the passage, writing that Onan both defrauded his late brother of his right and "no less cruelly than foully" committed this crime of contraception. Jeremy Taylor, an Anglican bishop of the seventeenth century, censured Onan who "did separate his act from its proper end."[4]

The story of Er and Onan served as the basis for condemnation in the Jewish tradition as well, but with interesting differences. Er, too, is presumed to have practised contraception, though his motives were obviously not those of Onan. He must have done so, says the Talmud, to avoid marring Tamar's fabled beauty with a pregnancy; or as a twelfth-century Bible commentator, Rabbi Joseph Bechor Shor, suggests alternatively: "Er didn't want the trouble of raising children, for there *are* such people who care only about their own convenience." But these and other homiletic interpretations aside, the point of the Onan story is clearly not about contraception in principle or even a particular means of contraception, but about a particular motive. Hence, the application of its pejorative teaching to means, such as coitus interruptus, in Jewish literature is by *remez* only, by intimation or homiletic suggestion only.

The clue to the story is the levirate context. Onan was given his late brother's wife for purposes of levirate mitzvah only. He had marital relations with her, but frustrated the real purpose. And—in answer to the question of why the punishment should have been so severe—he frustrated not just the real purpose but the only legitimate purpose that would save what he was doing from the category of a capital crime. The code of sexual ethics in Leviticus and Deuteronomy forbids marriage to a brother's widow on penalty of death, except for the special levirate circumstances—namely when the brother had left her childless, when marriage to her for this purpose becomes a mitzvah. Even "Noahides," the people of the generations before Sinai, were, from the Talmud's point of view, commanded concerning such incestuous marriages. Hence, the sin of Onan is a violation, by subterfuge, of a capital offense; his means of doing so serve, by intimation, to suggest something unseemly and objectionable in and of itself. It must, incidentally, be added that a contemporary rabbinic writer untypically resorts to a wholly naturalistic reading of the story, seeing in it neither violation of marriage law nor condign punishment by the wrath of God. "We do not have to assume childishly that a thunderbolt descended from heaven and struck Onan dead," he writes. The Bible is merely relating the *natural* effect of so unhealthy a practice as coitus interruptus: Onan suffered a heart attack from the nervous strain of it all![5]

But the idea of something unseemly and objectionable in and of itself does find full measure of censure in Talmud and, especially, in the Zohar, the mystic tradition. Here masturbation as well as coitus interruptus and other various forms of thwarting the natural manner of coitus are subsumed under "the act of Er and Onan," with consequent implications for the halakhic attitude toward contraception.

We return to our paradigmatic rabbi who cannot recommend abstinence to the couple for whom pregnancy would be hazardous, nor can he recommend that they place themselves in hazard. The remaining alternative is contraception; but what about the apparent onanism involved? The dilemma, of course, describes the premodern situation before oral contraceptives, such as the pill, entered the picture. The condom and similar means do entail onanism, hence the dilemma in much of the Responsa literature.

But if hazard threatens, then even the formidable objection of onanism must be set aside, and the dilemma resolved in favor of ongoing marital relations. It is highly significant that antiabstinence considerations are not overruled, but those of onanism are. In that famous talmudic source-passage, the Baraita of the Three Women, the various levels of interpretation all revolve around whether the three categories of women may or must, or may not or need not, practice contraception before, during or after, with this, that or the other kind of contraceptive principle. The clearly implied alternative is marital relations without contraception, never abstinence.

And there is even more to weigh down this side of the scale. Not only must the relational mitzvah of marital sex be added to the procreational, and not only must the ongoing frequency and inalienable nature of the mitzvah be considered, but so must the quality of the sexual relationship. This factor derives from still another mitzvah, having to do with a "draft deferment" for the new groom. Deuteronomy (24:5) says: "If a man takes a new wife, he should not go out to war. He should remain home for a year and rejoice [with] his wife whom he has married." The rabbis focused on the verb in this verse, *ve'simmach*, "rejoice." It confirmed to them that "rejoicing one's wife" is synonymous with proper marital relations. Indeed, they used the phrase *simchat ishto* as a synonym for such, and taught that the mitzvah is not fulfilled unless there is joy for the wife, that the quality of the mitzvah is no less a factor than its frequency. As the Talmud puts it generally (*Pesahim* 72b): "A man must cause his wife to rejoice in this matter of mitzvah."

This qualitative consideration, by the way, figured in the details of rabbinic Responsa on birth control. After having concluded that contraception is indicated in a specific situation, the next question was the kind of device or method to be used. Since some devices by their very nature deny to the woman the natural gratification of physical propinquity, they would thus deprive the act of its requisite qualitative dimension. Some Responsa, accordingly, refer to the phrase in Genesis ". . . and cleave unto his wife, and they shall be as one flesh" to make the point. In order that the sexual mitzvah be fulfilled properly, they must be "as one flesh," with no occlusive or impedimental barriers to separate them.[6] Orally ingested contraceptives, such as the pill, are therefore preferable to other devices; they are neither onanistic nor do they diminish the physical gratification.

A standard commentary to the Talmud, that of Maharsha (Rabbi Shlomo Edels) of the seventeenth century, gives us the conclusion of the discussion on the purpose of the sexual mitzvah. Like such discussions in other cultures before and after, coordinate and subordinate purposes are stated. In the Jewish system, says Maharsha, sex has a twofold coequal purpose: to enable procreation and to "fulfill her desire." Hence, "rejoicing one's wife" is a mitzvah in its own right, and the rabbi must apply it to the scale as well.

Maharsha's phrase, "to fulfill her desire," however, has another source, one that leads to another discussion, both theological and exegetical. His source is Genesis 3:16, in the context of the "curse of Eve." This is very much a part of the classic Christian doctrine of original sin and of the punishment therefor visited upon the descendants of Adam and Eve. In the Talmud and Jewish tradition, both the sin and its punishment have a different role entirely.

The verse setting forth the punishment for Eve is twofold. It reads: "In pain shalt thou give birth, and unto thy husband will be thy desire, but he will rule over you." To take the second curse first (and return later to "in pain shalt thou give birth"), the Talmud analyzes its meaning (*Eiruvin* 100a). What does "unto thy husband will be thy desire" mean? It means that a woman will have a sexual desire, at least like that of her husband. So what's the curse? The curse is in the next clause: ". . . but he will rule over you." Since the male is more aggressive and brazen, and the female more coy and refined—either by nature or by nurture, either biologically or culturally—the male feels free to initiate sexual activity more readily than does the female, though her desire is equally there! This imbalance is awkward, painful, a "curse." If that is the case, says the Talmud in this passage, then it is a mitzvah for the husband to spare his wife this curse, this awkwardness, and to initiate sexual relations when he observes her to be desirous but too shy or refined to say so. Hence, says the Talmud, and the Codes of Law follow: When a man notices that his wife is desirous, then he now has a conjugal mitzvah over and above the standard frequency. He should save her, so to speak, from this "curse" by initiating sexual relations in keeping with her perceived desire.[7]

The theological implications are profound. It means that Eve's descendants are not supposed to endure any curse because of her; her sin does not attach to them, neither does the punishment. It is, rather, one's mitzvah to spare her any such consequences.

But first it is worth dwelling on other implications. Morton Hunt, in *The Natural History of Love*, tells us that the presence of sexual desire in women was not acknowledged until recently. Until the end of the nineteenth century, he writes, one would be accused of "casting vile aspersions on womankind" if he suggested that women have sexual desire or, worse, experience sexual pleasure. While this may have been true in the Western world, in Jewish culture and tradition both sexual desire and sexual pleasure of women are not only acknowledged but made into a religious concern for men. This is illustrated by Maharsha's statement above, which makes explicit the talmudic teaching: "To fulfill her desire" is one of the two purposes of the sexual mitzvah.

But if this is associated with the verse in Genesis, why was the concept, at least, of female sexual desire not acknowledged more widely in the Western world? The answer may lie in a scrutiny of Bible translations through history. In the second century, St. Jerome gave the phrase a more neutral rendering. For *el ishekh t'shukatekh*, he translated "Unto thy husband wilt thou turn," rather than "Unto thy husband will be thy desire." This rendering was followed in most subsequent versions, with the notable exception of that of Gregory, a sixteenth-century monk, who came closer to the original Hebrew and restored the phrase to the traditional Jewish meaning. Perhaps because of "cultural lag" the notion did not take hold until the late nineteenth century.

More to the point: anesthesia was demonstrated in Massachusetts General Hospital in 1840. When it occurred to doctors there to use it to relieve the pain of childbirth, strong objections were heard from religious, notably Catholic, circles. How can anesthesia be used for such purposes, allowing us to fly in the face of an explicit biblical command to "give birth in pain"? In France in the nineteenth century, two women were condemned to death for administering or accepting anesthesia in childbirth.[8] The doctors then turned to the rabbis, adherents of the "Old Testament," for their position on the matter. They responded, in keeping with rabbinic understanding of the Bible generally, that to "give birth in pain" is not a command but a curse, and that it is our mitzvah to spare the woman any such curse with whatever means we have.

This teaching was obviously a latter-day application of the above talmudic treatment of the theology of that verse. Just as the Talmud had declared it the husband's mitzvah to spare her the purported curse of being less sexually aggressive than he, it becomes our mitzvah to spare her the curse implied earlier in the verse as well. "Give birth in pain" is not a commandment, nor is it counted as such in any of the lists of commandments, 613 or otherwise. Further, there is no reason to assume that the guilt or punishment of Eve should accrue to her descendants. But commandments to be concerned with preventing pain to women and enhancing their welfare occur throughout the Torah. The rabbis accordingly made it emphatically clear that use of anesthesia—providing it is both physically and psychologically indicated—is not only permissible but desirable.

The rabbis of our day had even more to go on in talmudic sources for their position on the question of anesthesia. There is a striking narrative in the Talmud (*Yevamot* 65a) in which the wife of one of the talmudic greats, Rabbi Hiyya, had suffered from unusual childbirth pain and thus wanted to avoid further births. A kind of contraceptive was available that was actually a sterilizing potion (*kos shel ikkarin*). She wanted to take advantage of it but first had to consult rabbinic authority. Fearing her husband would not be impartial in so personal a matter, she left her house through the back door, disguised herself, and came in through the front door, appearing as a stranger asking a religious question. "Who," she asked, "is responsible to fulfill the mitzvah of procreation, the man or the woman?" "The man," Rabbi Hiyya answered. "Well, then," she continued, "I experience great pain in childbirth. Am I permitted to take a sterilizing potion to prevent future pregnancies and be spared this severe pain?" "Yes," he said. "Since it is not your responsibility, you are entitled to save yourself such pain by taking the potion." "Thank you," she said, went out and around to the back entrance, removed her disguise, came back into the house and identified herself as his recent questioner. "The answer remains," he said, "but I wish you had waited to give birth just one more time."

For our purposes, the point of this story is that it did not occur to Rabbi Hiyya that she must endure severe childbearing pain. Not only did he not invoke the Genesis verse, the sin of Eve having nothing to do with her, but he regarded childbirth pain, when especially severe, as sufficient warrant for sterilization; the husband's mitzvah of procreation cannot be fulfilled at the cost of her "great pain."

The story has an echo in the nineteenth century, in the Responsa works of the great *Hatam Sofer*, Rabbi Moses Sofer (d. 1839).[9] The question of sterilization was asked again on behalf of a woman who experienced unusual pain in childbirth. Hatam Sofer replied that the question had already been clearly answered in the Talmud—except, of course, that polygamy was theoretically possible in those days. Which means that Rabbi Hiyya's answer presupposed that the husband of a woman who took the sterilizing potion could always fulfill his mitzvah or desire for children through another wife. But now since polygamy has been officially banned by Rabbenu Gershom in the tenth century—it was rare in Western countries anyway, but now formally forbidden—Rabbi Hiyya's advice must be reconsidered. If the present questioner does make herself sterile it will be unfair to the husband who no longer has the alternative of polygamy. Therefore, says Hatam Sofer, let her first secure her husband's consent. But then, he continues, if the husband refuses consent, let her do so anyway, because his desire for children, or to fulfill the mitzvah, cannot be accomplished at the cost of her great pain. As to her own desire to have children, on the teaching that a woman's fulfillment comes from having children, that her glory is in building the next generation, Hatam Sofer comes down on the side of the individual woman: "She cannot be asked to build the world by destroying herself"—assuming the pain in her case to have been severe, even "destructive." The fact is that Rabbi Sofer did not invoke Genesis 3:16, nor any concept of need or merit in suffering. Anesthesia, it may be recalled, was made available in 1840; he died in 1839.

To return finally to our composite rabbi with his figurative scales: The balance is overwhelmingly weighted in favor of ongoing marital relations even if nonprocreative, and even if onanism is ultimately unavoidable, as against exposing oneself to hazard or choosing abstinence. This says so much for the spiritual-physical equilibrium in this area of human and religious life.

There is yet another key principle in marital relations, which also figures on the scale of values in answering specific religious-legal questions and characterizes the general attitude to marriage. It is the lovely concept of *sh'lom bayyit*—"domestic tranquillity," or harmony of the home—and it raises the ideal of peaceful relations at home above even the ideal of truth.

The Talmud bases its doctrine of *sh'lom bayyit* on a perceived discrepancy between what Sarah said of Abraham and what God reported to Abraham. Sarah had said, "How can I give birth, seeing that my husband is old?" When God speaks to Abraham, he puts it: "Why did Sarah ask 'How can I give birth, seeing that I am old?'" The rabbis note that Sarah had attributed the age problem to her husband, but God "modified" her words. Had he reported them exactly, there would have been resentment of Sarah by Abraham; there would have been a loss of *sh'lom bayyit*. We learn from this that if even God, Whose seal is Truth, can "modify" the story in order to preserve *sh'lom bayyit* between husband and wife, how much more should the rest of us modify and subordinate truth to peace, to peace between husband and wife and between man and his fellow-men.[10]

Actually, the biblical source of the teaching for the Talmud is elsewhere, in the legal portion of the Book of Numbers, where the rite of the *Sotah* is described. There we are told that if a man harbors suspicions about his wife's fidelity, the suspicions can be allayed through the Ordeal of Jealousy. The ordeal requires, among other things, that words of oath be written on parchment, then washed off into a potion that she would drink. If she proves guilty, her stomach distends and her thighs descend; if she is innocent, nothing of this kind happens, and the husband must abandon his suspicions.

This ordeal has, incidentally, been interpreted by modern Bible scholars in a new light. The use of the word ordeal is not actually warranted, they claim, because ordeals are intended to show guilt, not innocence. In the ordeal by fire, for example, the victim has a hot firebrand placed on his tongue; if his tongue burns, he is adjudged guilty; if it miraculously shows no effect, then he is adjudged innocent. In an ordeal by water, the victim is tied to weights. Again, if he is weighed down and sinks, he is guilty; if he nonetheless floats, he is found innocent. Ordeals, in other words, typically judge guilt, not innocence; only by some miracle could the victim emerge unscathed.

By contrast, the "ordeal" of the Sotah is intended to prove her innocence, not her guilt. The "bitter waters" could produce no adverse effect, except perhaps a psychological one, like that of a polygraph. A guilty conscience could cause the physiological effects listed in the text—which probably describes a miscarriage—but a clear conscience would leave her totally unaffected by the drink. Hence the "ordeal," says a recently published study, was a favor to the woman; it would help her dispel unfounded suspicions.[11]

This is essentially the talmudic view of the matter. The solemn adjuration, written on parchment, included the name of God. Accordingly, when the question was raised in the Talmud about "erasing the Name" as part of the procedure, the answer underscored the supreme importance of *sh'lom bayyit*. The ordeal called for the oath to be "erased into" the waters which she would subsequently drink. How could God allow His Name to be desecrated by erasure, when we are taught elsewhere that this is forbidden? Only, is the answer, because the ideal of amity between husband and wife is so precious that God allowed His Name to be dissolved in the service thereof, in removing suspicion and restoring harmony. In no fewer than five instances in the Talmud is this point made, derived from the same source. Responsa writers, too, relay the idea in discussing practical questions and resolving legal conflicts in marital situations: "Since the Divine Name was permitted to be erased when the purpose of restoring confidence and peace between husband and wife was at issue [in the biblical rite], how much more so may such and such be done to preserve or restore that peace."[12]

Now, this sublime concept of *sh'lom bayyit* is a spiritual rather than a physical one. Yet the blend is seen here too. First, it must be noted that preserving *sh'lom bayyit* becomes a legal factor in some questions of contraception and abortion. When the mitzvah of *p'ru ur'vu* has been minimally fulfilled, further procreation need not be undertaken if it would serve as a strain on the marriage; that is, if *sh'lom bayyit* is threatened. And while economic considerations are not admissible as a warrant for abortion, a threat to this spiritual concept may be.

A more telling indication of the spiritual-physical blend is the Talmud's use of this same phrase in the purely physical sense. The decline of one's sexual powers is there (*Shabbat* 152a) described as—a decline in *sh'lom bayyit*. The physical partakes of the spiritual, and the spiritual has its very physical dimension.

The spiritual facets of physical marriage are many. There is the custom, not uncommon even today, whereby the bride and groom fast on their wedding day until after the ceremony. The time before the ceremony becomes their own private Yom Kippur, to heighten the sense of threshold, of beginning a new life with high resolve.

The spiritual elements of restraint and of purity are introduced into the marriage relationship by an elaborate system of Niddah laws. Intimate relations are proscribed during the time of menstruation and until after cleansing and purification in the waters of Mikveh. The Talmud elaborates the details of Niddah separation, defines the specifics of the purification process, then comments on the nonphysical value of the regimen: The enforced cyclical separation prevents the opposite of abstinence—easy availability; it means that reunion after purification will give the relationship the freshness of a new, recurrent honeymoon.

Access to one's wife can be forbidden even at times other than Niddah. The legal and moral codes have much to say against approaching one's wife when both he and she are not in harmony. He may not, for example, approach her when he is intoxicated, because no conscious love can be present; nor in a state of enmity, for such is harlotry rather than conjugality;

or when divorce has been decided on, for similar reasons. Perhaps alone among the cultures of the world, Jewish law does recognize the charge of rape in the marital context. A husband clearly has no automatic right to approach his wife; they must be physically and emotionally in harmony; otherwise he is guilty of rape. Generally, the wife's desires are primary and take precedence over his. (The popular medieval compendium *Sefer Hasidim* [*The Book of the Pious*], therefore regards one as especially fortunate if his wife's wishes happen to coincide with his own in sexual matters. Of him does Proverbs 18:22 speak when it says "He who has found a wife has found good, and has obtained favor of the Lord.")[13] Jewish sexual ethics can be generally described as a concern for the other rather than a matter of self-indulgence.

The famous thirteenth-century text called *Iggeret haKodesh* (*Epistle of Holiness*), in its chapter "On the Quality of the Act," puts it this way: "Therefore engage her first in conversation that puts her heart and mind at ease and gladdens her. Thus your mind and intent will be in harmony with hers. Speak words which arouse her to passion, union, love, desire and eros—and words which elicit attitudes of reverence for God, piety and modesty.... Never may you force her, for in such union the Divine Presence cannot abide. Your intent is then different from hers, and her mind not in accord with yours. Quarrel not with her, nor strike her; as our Sages taught 'Just as a lion tramples and devours and has no shame, so a boorish man strikes and copulates and has no shame.' Rather win her over with words of graciousness and seductiveness..."[14]

All this is part of the ethic, alongside considerations of the health factor, in sexual expression. Even the austere Maimonides, who enumerated the ill effects of overindulgence in sex as well as food, acknowledged the beneficial effects of moderate sexual release. The most expansive and well-nigh lyrical statement of the health value of conjugal relations for the man was offered by Rabbi Jacob Emden (d. 1776). Following earlier writers on the subject, he expounded on the substantial advantages to the body, to the disposition and even to the soul, of appropriate sexual expression. Interesting for our theme of the blending of the physical and spiritual, Emden's formulation appears in his prayer-book compendium, in the section on Friday Evening customs and practices.[15] Since the Talmud (*K'tubot* 62b) had declared the Sabbath as particularly right for conjugal relations—because, in Rashi's words, that is the "time of pleasure, rest, and physical well-being," and, in the words of both Iggeret ha-Kodesh and a later work called *M'norat ha-Maor*, the Sabbath is spiritual and lends one a *n'shamah y'teirah* (extra dimension of soul)—the idea is carried forward by Emden's words and placement thereof. Sexual expression must be considerate, but it is both healthful and spiritual. The latter stands in contrast, it must be said, to the position taken by some marriage manuals circulating in the Middle Ages that disapproved of sex, even for the best motives, on days holy on the Christian calendar. The conjugal-physical was never regarded here as inimical to the spiritual. It is incompatible only with Yom Kippur and, by extension, other fast days or the Shivah period of mourning, when indulgence in physical pleasure is itself proscribed.

The health factor, then, blends with the spiritual and moral considerations in marital sex, though these latter are primary. This applies as well to illicit sex or promiscuity, where one would expect a threat of venereal disease to figure prominently in exhortations to proper conduct. Instead, very little mention of such reasons for sexual probity can be found in the vast moralistic literature of Judaism on the subject. The motives invoked are always those of holiness, of respect for personhood, of the intrinsic indecency of harlotry. Departures from probity are legislated against not because of physical ills or crimes they may lead to, but because of their moral consequences for mind, attitude and spirit. The crimes they constitute are not "victimless"; they compromise fidelity and modesty, and trivialize the holy and personal.

The spiritual-physical balance is not easy to come by, but its importance in both the problem and the solution of sexual morality is highlighted in a different way by a contemporary writer. In his *Crisis and Faith*, Rabbi Eliezer Berkowitz addresses the causes of malaise in modern society.[16] We are unhappy participants in the sexual revolution because, he declares, we have lost this balance. Pauline Christianity emphasized the soul at the expense of the body, and individuals chose celibacy and abstinence or guilt in indulgence. Then came psychology, admonishing us to cast off guilt and cease the outrage against the body, which we have in common with other animals. To stifle the demands of the body, it was claimed, is to invite neuroses and actual illness. Individuals followed the new wisdom and its implications; they gave free rein to the body's imperious impulses, but at the expense of the moral or even the social and human. This is an outrage now against our spiritual nature, leading to undiagnosed but certain malaise.

Not intended to be either angel or animal, we find our way most wholesomely on this earth in the body-soul hyphenation. Health in the best sense comes from the balanced deference to both physical and spiritual components of our being.

· 8 ·

Procreation

The Jewish tradition has what today would be called a pronatalist thrust. Procreation is a positive mitzvah, enumerated in the list of commandments and given pride of place at the top thereof. A medieval summarizing text, one that organizes the commandments and elucidates them, states: Its purpose is that the world be populated. This is a great mitzvah, because through it, all others—which were given to humans and not to angels—may be fulfilled.[1]

Pride of place comes from early narratives of Genesis, but not necessarily from "be fruitful and multiply" in Genesis 1:28. As a participant in the Vatican Council reminded us, "The world has changed much since Adam and Eve, alone in the Garden, were told to multiply." Most commentators interpret that verse as for purposes "of blessing only," pointing to the same phrase a few verses earlier (Gen. 1:22) in connection with fish and fowl, which can be the object of blessing but not of commandment. An added dimension of commandment for humans was confirmed by later verses— one to the sons of Noah after the Flood (Gen. 9:1, 9) and to Jacob (Gen. 35:11).

A medieval commentator (Isaac Abravanel, d. 1508) sees the command rather than blessing as necessary because man, created in the image of God, might seek to devote himself entirely to the spiritual and intellectual and neglect the material and physical. Hence the commandment to instruct him that the preservation of the physical world is also his duty. A commentator of our own day, Rabbi Meir Me'iri, points out that only man is aware of the consequences of his sexual activity. He might seek to avoid the attendant responsibilities of childbirth while indulging his sexual drive; hence the commandment added in the case of man, over the similar blessing for fish and fowl. And, to cite still another comment: Throughout Genesis 1, "The Lord saw that it was good" is repeated after each element of creation was brought forth. But when man was created, the Lord said "It is *not good* that man should be alone." Only that which can endure is good; if man does not procreate he will not endure.[2]

Nor will God Himself endure. "He who does not engage in procreation is as if he diminished the Divine Image, as it says: "Whoso sheds the blood of man, by man shall his blood be shed, for in the image of God has He created man" (Gen. 9:6), which is immediately followed by "be fruitful and multiply" (9:7). Or, the later verse introduces the Lord Who will be "thy God and [that] of thy descendants after thee" (17:7). But "if there are no descendants after thee," demands the Talmud, "upon whom will the Divine Presence rest? Upon sticks and stones?" Without human descendants, there is no one to worship God. Without the physical body, there is no soul.

In spelling out the details of this commandment, the rabbis require that a couple at least replace itself; that is, that a couple give birth to at least a son and a daughter. Having several sons or several daughters, then, does not yet fulfill the commandment. But "grandchildren are like children," so parents of children of one gender only can be comforted they have a second chance in the grandchildren! But even having one of each gender remains a minimum only; sticking to that minimum, says *Tosafot*, could well lead to national extinction.[3] Infant mortality or uncertainty about whether the offspring themselves will be viable persons or parents require, say the rabbis, that more than the minimum be sired.

The rabbinic dimension of the mitzvah was called, in brief, *la-shevet* or *la-erev*. The first comes from the verse in Isaiah (45:18): "Not for void did He create the world, but for habitation [*la-shevet*] did He form it." The second is from Ecclesiastes (11:6): "In the morning sow thy seed, and in the evening [*la-erev*] do not withhold thy hand [from continuing to sow], for you know not which will succeed, this or that, or whether they shall both alike be good."[4]

The Sefer [scroll of the] Torah is a most sacred object. Laws govern its proper care and under what circumstances it may be sold. It may be sold only to finance education in the Torah or to dower a bride, to make possible a marriage where procreation—even the rabbinic dimensions of *la-shevet* and *la-erev*—has yet to be fullfilled.

It goes without saying that attitudes to procreation were not shaped or nurtured through law alone. Abraham protests to God, "What canst Thou give me, seeing that I go childless?" (Gen. 15:2). The anguish of the barren woman is a recurrent theme in the Bible and beyond. The most cherished blessing, on the other hand, is fecundity, which is exemplified idyllically in the Psalmist's image of one whose "wife is a fruitful vine" and whose "children are as olive plants around the table" and whose ultimate satisfaction is the sight of "children [born] to thy children" (Ps. 128).

Historical circumstances of frequent massacres and forced conversions, with their decimation of Jewish communities, served to elicit compensatory tendencies and to strengthen the procreative desire. The people's will to replenish its depleted ranks gave added dimension to the instinctive yearning for offspring. This contrasts, for example, with the antiprocreational stand, born of despair, taken by the first-century Gnostics, the fifth-century Manichees or the twelfth-century Cathars, who taught and lived by the teaching that procreation is to be avoided in an evil world.[5]

In the face of a precarious future, procreation is essentially an act of faith. When medical considerations make pregnancy dangerous, there is the inclination to be equally trusting. Even normal pregnancy is by definition dangerous, and these normal risks are incurred by necessity and desire. But with real risk, in especially hazardous situations, the rabbis legislated against fulfilling one commandment while ignoring the other commandment, to "take good heed of yourselves."

A technicality in Jewish law places the responsibility for procreation on the man and not the woman. This may have its basis in the theoretical permissibility of polygamy, or polygyny, as opposed to polyandry, whereby a man could have more than one wife. Each wife could defer responsibility to the other. The sex-role difference is associated with the verse "Be fruitful and multiply and fill the earth and conquer it"—that he, being the more aggressive, the conqueror, must "worry about" procreation; whereas she, the less aggressive, should not have to "go seeking in the marketplace." These reasons are improved upon by the suggestion of a recent Bible commentator, Rabbi Meir Simchah of Dvinsk (d. 1927): Both the pain and the risk of childbearing are borne by the woman, not the man. Since the Torah is not only fair but "Its ways are ways of pleasantness and all its paths are peace" (Prov. 3:17), the Torah could not in fairness command a woman to undergo pain and risk. This must be her choice.[6] For the man, however, who is exposed to neither pain nor risk, there is the command and the responsibility to fulfill the command.

With so pronatalist a general and specific tradition, the Jewish response has been understandably affirmative to new reproductive techniques, such as in-vitro fertilization. In some public discussions, these test-tube-assisted conceptions were opposed on principle: How can you violate natural law, or deviate from the natural process, whereby husband and wife, unassisted,

see to the conception and gestation of the embryo? In one of the early sym-
posia on the subject, I pointed out that (a) we have no problem with
natural law. Jewish philosophy has no concept of natural law in this sense.
We do not worship nature nor do we regard its laws as knowable and un-
breakable.

On the contrary, the process of creation is ongoing, and we seek to be
"partners with God" in conquering and controlling nature. Hence we ap-
plaud efforts to dam the rivers and prevent flooding, to use lightning rods,
or even air-conditioners, to overcome the tyranny of natural elements. We
even circumcise infant males rather than stand back and declare nature
perfect as such. The conclusion of the creation narrative in Genesis is
recited ceremonially at the Friday Evening Sabbath Meal, when the day is
sanctified by *Kiddush*. We thus sanctify the Sabbath which was ordained
at a point in creation when God had, in the literal translation, "ceased
from His work which He had created to do." "Created to do"? What does
that mean? the rabbis ask. It means that God created much yet to be done,
much for us to do now that we are here on earth to be partners in the continuation of the creative process.[7]

Hence, giving nature a little help when, for example, Fallopian tubes are
blocked, by circumventing this impediment through use of the Petri dish,
is quite acceptable, even meritorious. Furthermore, (b) it should be remembered that we have already "improved upon" nature in the very institution of marriage. Man is not naturally monogamous; primitives used to
mate indiscriminately. Religion and civilization have advanced beyond all
this by instituting marriage and known paternity. Most important, (c) the
desire of a woman for offspring is a deeply human one, and helping her
realize this desire is a positively human deed. As long as we can safeguard
against abuse, it is a mitzvah to resort, if necessary, to laboratory assistance
to help bring about this desired end.

In-vitro fertilization, however, has been superseded in some quarters by
the in-vivo method. Having the advantage of avoiding surgery—for the
fertilized ovum can then be lavaged out and implanted in the womb of
another—this procedure helps the woman who can conceive but not carry.
But then the question of maternity is raised: Who is the real mother?

In the Talmud's imagery, "There are three partners in the birth of the
human child"—the father, the mother and God. The mother actually gives
more. The genetic endowment of the father is matched both by the mother's
genetic endowment, the ovum, and by her gestational environment, the
womb. The question now is, if these two contributions are divided between
two women, one supplying the ovum and the other the womb, which one

is the mother? Moreover, in the case of surrogate mothers, where both of these contributions are offered by a client to her sponsor, what maternal claim accrues to the sponsor?

Even these ultramodern phenomena have their precedents in scripture. Rachel and Leah had their own children, but before and in between these births, they "sponsored" children through their handmaidens Bilhah and Zilpah. These handmaidens, as well as Hagar in Abraham's day, were prototypes of surrogate mothers. But they were free of the sociological problems that complicate the picture today. The "surrogates" did not have a change of heart and insist on keeping the babies, nor did the sponsors renege because the babies were not up to their expectations. Also, there was no financial arrangement. Safeguards need to be set up against these or other complications or abuses, so that they might be available in the absence of the "natural" alternative. England's Warnock Commission, in its report of July 1984, recommended against surrogate-mother arrangements because the potential of abuse is so great. Its Chief Rabbi, I. Jakobovitz, endorsed the verdict, adding: "To use another person as 'incubator' and then take from her the child she carried and delivered, for a fee, is a revolting degradation of maternity and an affront to human dignity." In America, the Michigan Court of Appeals in 1981 viewed the surrogate arrangement as a form of forbidden "baby bartering," although supporters maintain the payment is for "services" rather than for the baby, which belonged to the sponsors to begin with.

The question of maternity can be resolved in favor of the *sponsoring* mother by arguing that the genetic, as opposed to the gestational, contribution is the dynamic one with the all-important genetic code. Also, the donated zygote can already be said to be a nascent being, with the identity of the child already intact. From another standpoint, the first mother's role is not replaceable by technology, while the host mother's is; the gestation could conceivably be done in the laboratory.

On the other hand, maternity can be argued for the *host* mother on these grounds: A transplanted organ becomes an integral part of the body of the recipient, which means that the recipient of an ovarian transplant becomes the mother. Also, the host mother gives both nurture and gestation to the embryo. As a Congressional committee was told in August 1984, "The biological fact is that the gestational mother has contributed more of herself to the child than the genetic mother, and therefore has a greater biological investment and interest in it." Moreover, the legal presumption in favor of the host mother "gives the child and society certainty of identification at the time of birth, which is a protection for both mother and child." If looked at from the point of view of the mother's "sacrifice," it must be added, then nine months of responsible nurture is a far greater "gift" than the surrender of an ovum, entitling her far more clearly to acknowledgment of parenthood.

Too much "on the one hand" and "on the other hand"? Accordingly, Israeli hospitals, where such in-vivo fertilization has taken place, now list *both* mothers on the birth certificate. For the first time in history, while we find our way through the mind-boggling implications of new developments in reproductive technology, babies are recorded as having two mothers. Two maternal relationships, like that of mother and father, may exist simultaneously.

Of course, Jewish law would never sanction recourse to any such methods merely to spare one the inconvenience of pregnancy and childbearing, and certainly not in order to insure some package of genetic characteristics, such as blue eyes or tall stature. But where there is no natural alternative, these resourceful ways of bringing about the desideratum become acceptable. Enabling a woman to fulfill the maternal yearning, or a couple to fulfill the mitzvah, is itself a mitzvah.

In medical ethics committee sessions, analysis has made explicit what is implicit in Jewish legal tradition. We have declared "barrenness" to be an "illness," a loss of normal health. Accordingly, all the principles of setting aside ritual and other laws of the Torah prevail here, too: The same may and should be done to help overcome infertility as would be done for any other pathological condition.

Before in-vitro or in-utero fertilization was a gleam in anyone's eye, assistance to procreation was found in artificial insemination, either of a husband's immotile sperm (AIH), or of a donor's sperm (AID) when the husband was infertile as well as impotent. These procedures bring in tow a different set of halakhic and moral problems, though AIH much less so.

Problems in connection with artificial insemination by the husband involve mainly the procurement of the semen, that is the avoidance of onanism. Also, the unwitting or deliberate admixture of the semen of another, to increase fertility strength, is unacceptable. Done properly, the procedure is a welcome solution to some infertility cases.

But AID represents the greater number of problems. Some rabbinic authorities declare the process adulterous and the offspring illegitimate. Others remind us that adultery is a conscious violation of the marriage vow by illicit intimacy, none of which takes place in this clinical procedure; hence no adultery or illegitimacy can be associated with artificial insemination by donor. Nonetheless, it does sever the human, family bond and it does conceal paternity, an important consideration in Jewish law. When the children grow they may unwittingly marry their siblings, meaning that unknown paternity has led to the grave sin of incest.[8]

Adoption, then, might seem the far better alternative, though the objection to unknown paternity applies here, too. Hence the identity of natural parents should be knowable to the child or to a readily accessible friend, to avoid the incest contingency. In the opinion of one psychological school of thought, adoption is preferable because it avoids resentment by the husband. If his wife had to be artificially inseminated by another, the child will bear her genetic endowment, which is a plus; but it leaves the husband out entirely, which is a minus. When the child is adopted, neither parent has genetic input, which is a minus; but it eliminates resentment or jealousy, or a reminder of the husband's disproportionate inadequacy, which is a plus.

None of the medically resourceful alternatives would be chosen, or permitted to be chosen, when conception and birth in the normal way are possible. An additional consideration for this point of view is the concept of lineage, an important one in Jewish tradition. To know and identify one's ancestors, and hopefully to seek to give them immortality by advancing their righteous aspirations, lends another spiritual dimension to one's own life and places it in a larger context of significance. Hence the custom of naming a child after a grandparent, giving a second chance to the ancestor and an inspiration to the descendant.

Eugenics, in the sense of choosing a marriage partner with the well-being of the progeny in mind, is also found in talmudic counsel and legislation.[9] A man is advised to choose a wife prudently, in accordance with her intellectual and moral virtues. Heredity as a eugenic principle takes its medical and legal model from halakhic rulings on circumcision. An infant whose two brothers died as a possible result of this operation may not be circumcised; he is deemed to have inherited the illness that proved fatal to his brothers. The same is then said of an infant whose two maternal cousins showed that weakness; that is, the statistical evidence yielded by two brothers from the same mother can also appear in two sisters of that mother (*Y'vamot* 64b). This reflects an early recognition that hemophilia is transmitted through maternal lineage, a significant eugenic discovery.

This in turn led to the first eugenic edict in any social or religious system. The statistical or presumptive evidence of adverse hereditary factors occasioned the ruling against marriage into a family of epileptics or lepers or, by extension, a similar disease. But while one view in the Talmud attributes the problem to physical characteristics of the marriage partner, another views it as the result of bad luck. In another context (*Mishnah, Eduyot* II, 9) we are told that a father bequeathes to his son "looks, strength, riches, and length of days"; again the commentators differ as to whether the apparent bequeathing is hereditary or a matter of influence or reward.

A related matter of eugenics begins with the Talmud's recommendation that one seek his sister's daughter as a bride. This is in the interests of fulfilling the injunction to "love one's wife as much as himself and to honor her more than himself," the idea being that his care for his wife will be the more tender due to his affection for his own sister. But in the thirteenth century, Rabbi Judah the Pious left a testamentary charge to his family against marriage with a niece, on the grounds that it bore adverse genetic consequence. His stature gave legal standing to his ruling. Considerations of social or hereditary factors that require, say, premarital blood testing are certainly endorsed by talmudic legislation.

The birth of a child is, of course, a blessing and a joyous occasion. In keeping with ritual purity considerations, however, the birthing mother suffers impurity for a period specified by the Bible, after which time she brought an offering at the altar, when the Temple still stood on its ancient site. The reason for the impurity has to do only with the physical discharges accompanied by childbirth, hence the offering at the completion of the period. The Talmud, incidentally, offers an additional reason, one with interesting psychological insight and with some bearing on what was said above. The Talmud's explanation is: We must presume that there is something for which the childbearing woman wants to atone, and the offering is her atonement. What would she be atoning for? Most likely, when labor or childbirth was painful, she took a vow never to become pregnant again, never to find herself in such a situation again. When the birth was completed and she saw the smiling infant, she hardly remembered either the vow or the pain of the circumstances that brought it about. Now, knowing only the joy of having the child, she has forgotten the vow and also the need to have it formally annulled. For this she needs to bring a sin-offering to the Temple!

Another point of interest in connection with postparturitional impurity is that the time period specified in the Bible differs for a boy child and a girl child: seven days for the male infant and fourteen for the female infant. A popular Bible commentary used in the synagogue, that of Britain's late Chief Rabbi I. H. Hertz, despairs of making sense of the difference and states simply: There is no satisfactory explanation of why the period of impurity is doubled for the female birth. The verse even misled Aristotle into making a groundless distinction *prenatally* in the formation of a male and female embryo. Actually, on the basis of a comment by the Talmud, the following may be suggested: Fourteen days should have been the normal period of impurity for all births. But since the next verse in the text reminds us that a male child is to be circumcised on the eighth day (Lev. 12:3), the impurity in this case must be halved in order to allow the mother to be present in purity for the occasion.

The pronatalist emphasis, then, is a pronounced one. It is balanced by concern for the woman's well-being, as we have seen, in a physical sense and otherwise. To this must be added another balancing consideration, as noted in the commentary *Akedat Yitzchak*, by Rabbi Isaac Arama of fifteenth-century Spain. The text in Genesis again has Rachel lament, in conversation with her husband Jacob, her failure so far to give birth. Jacob responds with apparent insensitivity: "What do you want from me? Am I in God's stead, Who denied you the fruit of the womb?" According to Arama, Jacob's perturbation was not insensitive but was an attempt to reassure Rachel that childbearing was not her only function. "Do I not love you just the same?" was his implied response, and Arama relayed the teaching, reminiscent of that of Hatam Sofer in another connection, that childbearing is not a woman's only function, and that she be beloved for herself.[10]

This became a legal issue on a different level, in consideration of the mishnaic statement that a man who has been married ten years to a barren wife is not "permitted to avoid fulfilling" the mitzvah of procreation any longer. Yet, with polygamy no longer an option, it was not an option for childlessness either. Rabbi Eliezer ben Joel HaLevi, an authority of the twelfth century, ruled out a bigamous solution to the problem of infertility or, worse, in the case of a sick wife. His Communal Council decreed: "Better that a [new] person should not be born than that this disgrace be perpetrated as a precedent for generations to come."[11] Nor is divorce a fair solution.

Rabbi Jacob Tannenbaum of Hungary sums it up in a Responsum at the end of the last century: "The Sages of previous generations have dealt at length with the matter and, it seems, could not find it in their hearts to permit in actual practice divorce against her will or the taking of a second wife, because of childlessness."[12] He adds the ethical observation that since this has now become standard procedure, a woman enters marriage on the understanding that she is not subject to unilateral divorce due to barrenness—and for a husband to act otherwise would be a breach of that understanding. Indeed, another rabbi had earlier relayed the suggestion that such a breach would be a violation of Leviticus 25:17, "Ye shall not wrong one another." This verse is applied by the Talmud especially to one's own wife, who may be more "sensitive to hurt."

Should, then, divorce by mutual consent be morally required in order to fulfill the procreative mitzvah? An answer, and a value judgment, is offered by a late Midrash that tells a beautiful story wherein "true love" prevails in the end. The Midrash, incidentally, dates from the time when plural marriage was permitted even in practice. A couple had been married for more than ten years without having been blessed with offspring. Since the duty of procreation had yet to be fulfilled, they agreed to part. The rabbi sought but failed to dissuade them; so he bade them celebrate their separation, like their union, with a feast. In the midst of merriment and good sentiment, the husband asked his wife to take with her her most desired object from the home, as a token of his continuing love. When the husband awoke from his inebriated state, he found himself in her father's house. *He* was, she said, the most precious treasure to her anywhere. They lived together "happily ever after."[13]

· 9 ·

This Matter of Abortion

The moral and political debate on the subject of this chapter continues unabated after several decades of modern discussion and analysis. Ultimate answers remain elusive, but several issues within the larger discussion can indeed be clarified.

Abortion played a major role in the 1984 political campaigns, as if the Supreme Court decision in January 1973 had resolved nothing at all. The right to take advantage of the Court's permissive ruling is itself the subject of debate, with efforts being launched to remove that right by constitutional amendment.

Six months before that historic Court decision, the legislature of the State of New York was among the first to abolish on its own any legal obstacles to abortion. Six months before that, NOW, the National Organization for Women, not anticipating such a turn of events, took New York State to court to have it enjoined to remove the antiabortion statute from its books. I was called to testify on behalf of NOW, but the exchange took the following unexpected form:

The attorney put the question to me: "Do you agree that the laws against abortion in New York State interfere with your freedom of religion, with your right to practice the rabbinate as you see fit?" Surprised by my reply in the negative, she demanded: "What do you mean, 'no'? I read your book *Birth Control in Jewish Law* and I got the distinct impression you would say 'yes.'"

"You must first answer a prior question," I replied. "Namely, is abortion murder? If it is murder, then you cannot talk about freedom of religion. There is no freedom of religion in the face of murder. To take an example, the Bible tells us that the ancient Canaanites used to practice child sacrifice. They would take a born child and sacrifice it on the altar. The Torah calls this an abomination and forbids us to do it. Now, what if these Canaanites or their modern counterparts were to come to America and wish to practice child sacrifice here, in the name of freedom of religion? Would we allow it? Of course not. If we forbid polygamy to the Mormons, we're certainly not going to permit murder to anyone on the grounds of religious freedom. But if abortion is not murder, then we can talk about it. Then I would say, yes, it does interfere with my ministry. Since Jewish law does not equate it with murder, there are circumstances under which Jewish law would permit, or even mandate, an abortion. But I am not at liberty to invoke any lenient rulings of Jewish law as long as the State law forbids it."

The attorney heaved a sigh of relief and pressed on to the next question: "Do you not agree that the State's law against abortion is a violation of women's rights, of the right of a woman to do with her body or her reproductive faculties as she sees fit?" Again I said "no," and again she was flustered. "What do you mean 'no'? Your book clearly implies that you would answer 'yes.'"

"Again I must say you have first got to answer the prior question. Is abortion murder? If it is, then you cannot talk about women's rights. There are no rights to murder. May a woman take a gun and shoot a one-year-old child or a ten- or twenty-year-old person, on the grounds that that person is the fruit of her womb? Of course not. But if the antiabortion people are right, then what happens after birth is equal to what happens before birth, and no woman has any more right to end a life then than later. So the right of a woman to her body or reproductive faculties is just not relevant, not applicable. But if abortion is not murder, then we can talk about it. Then I would say that the State's law does infringe on the rights of women. I would go much further and say that it infringes even more than you might think. Because in the Jewish legal-moral tradition on abortion, the woman's welfare plays an even greater role than NOW would claim. A principle in the Jewish view of the matter is *tza'ara d'gufah kadim*, that her welfare, avoidance of her pain, comes first.

"Accordingly," I continued, "maternal indications for abortion do count where fetal indications do not. It's not that the fetus has a right to be born or that the husband has a right to his progeny, but it's the welfare of the mother that is the first, and to some the only, consideration that warrants an abortion." The court trial proceeded as it did, but the points made above need now to be set forth.

Abortion is not murder, vociferous and repeated claims to the contrary notwithstanding. Abortion cannot be murder in Jewish law, because, as indicated above, murder is one of the three "cardinal" sins that require martyrdom. Rather than commit murder of the innocent, public idolatry or gross sexual immorality [adultery-incest], one has to surrender his own life in martyrdom. All the rest of the Torah is under the category of *ya'avor v'al ye-hareg*, "let one transgress rather than die," but not for murder of the innocent. Hence if abortion were declared murder, a mother would not be allowed to have an abortion even to save her life, which is obviously not the case.

There is—need it be stated?—no Commandment that reads "Thou shalt not kill." It reads, "Thou shalt not murder." The difference is in the circumstances. Killing is allowed in self-defense, in war, perhaps by a sentencing court, even in the case of a prowler. In these situations the victim is no longer innocent; he has forfeited his protection under the Commandment. He must, of course, do so consciously. He must have deliberately placed himself in a position of attack or threat in order to lose his protection. Another such category is that of *rodef*, the aggressor, who may be killed if that is the only way to stop his pursuit or aggression of a third party.

The Talmud considers defining the fetus as a *rodef*, an aggressor against its mother, and making that the reason why abortion to save the mother's life is permitted. (The idea entered the writings of St. Thomas Aquinas through its citation in the works of Maimonides.) But the Talmud proceeds to reject that reasoning on the obvious grounds that the fetus is not yet of responsible age to deliberately forfeit its protection against being murdered. The only valid grounds for permitting even therapeutic abortion is that murder is not involved because the fetus is not yet a human person.[1] Killing is admittedly involved, but not murder. Killing is the taking of life of, say, an animal or a chicken, or of a human who forfeits his protection by an act of aggression. And the difference between fetal life and human life is not determined by the biologist or the physician but by the metaphysician. It's the determination of the culture or the religion that declares not when life begins but when life begins to be human.

To trace the issues from the start, the abortion question in talmudic law revolves around the legal status of the embryo. For this the Talmud has a phrase, *ubbar yerekh immo*, which phrase is a counterpart of the Latin *pars viscerum matris*. That is, the fetus is deemed a "part of its mother," rather than an independent entity. This designation says nothing about the morality of abortion; rather, it defines ownership, for example, in the case of an embryo found in a purchased animal. As intrinsic to its mother's body, it belongs to the buyer. In the religious conversion of a pregnant woman, her unborn child is automatically included and requires no further ceremony. Nor does it have power of acquisition; gifts made on its behalf are not binding. These and similar points mean only that the fetus has no "juridical personality," but say nothing about the right of abortion. This turns rather on whether feticide is or is not homicide.[2]

The law of homicide in the Torah, in one of its formulations, reads: "*Makkeh ish . . .*" "He who smites a man . . ." (Ex. 21:12). Does this include any man, say a day-old child? Yes, says the Talmud, citing another text: ". . . *ki yakkeh kol nefesh adam*" "If one smite any *nefesh adam*" (Lev. 24: 17)—literally, any human person. (Whereas we may not be sure that the newborn babe has completed its term and is a *bar kayyama*, fully viable, until thirty days after birth, he is fully human from the moment of birth. If he dies before his thirtieth day, no funeral or *shivah* rites are applicable either. But active destruction of a born child of even doubtful viability is here definitely forbidden.)[3] The "any" (*kol*) is understood to include the day-old child, but the "*nefesh adam*" is taken to exclude the fetus in the womb. The fetus in the womb, says Rashi, classic commentator on the Bible and Talmud, is *lav nefesh hu*, not a person, until he comes into the world.[4]

Feticide, then, does not constitute homicide, and the basis for denying it capital-crime status in Jewish law—even for those rabbis who may have wanted to rule otherwise—is scriptural. Alongside the above text is another one in Exodus that reads: "If men strive, and wound a pregnant woman so that her fruit be expelled, but no harm befall [her], then shall he be fined as her husband shall assess . . . But if harm befall [her], then shalt thou give life for life" (21:22). The Talmud makes this verse's teaching explicit: Only monetary compensation is exacted of him who causes a woman to miscarry. Note also that though the abortion spoken of here is accidental, it contrasts with the homicide (of the mother) which is also accidental. Even unintentional homicide cannot be expiated by a monetary fine.[5]

This critical text, to begin with, has an alternative version in the Septuagint, the Greek translation of the Bible produced in Alexandria in the third pre-Christian century. A change of just one word there yields an entirely different statute on the subject. Professor Viktor Aptowitzer's essays analyze the disputed passage: The school of thought it represents he calls the Alexandrian school, as opposed to the Palestinian—that is, the talmudic—view set forth above. The word in question is *ason*, rendered here as "harm"; hence, "if [there be] harm, then shalt thou give life for life." The Greek renders *ason* as form, yielding something like: "If [there be] form, then shalt thou give life for life." The "life for life" clause is thus applied to fetus instead of mother *and* a distinction is made—as Augustine will formulate it

—betweeen *embryo informatus* and *embryo formatus*. For the latter, the text so rendered prescribes the death penalty.[6]

Among the Church Fathers, the consequent doctrine of feticide as murder was preached by Tertullian, in the second century, who accepted the Septuagint, and by Jerome in the fourth, who did not. Jerome's classic Bible translation renders the passage according to the Hebrew text accepted in the Church. The Didache, a handbook of basic Christianity for the instruction of converts from paganism, follows the Alexandrian teaching and specifies abortion as a capital crime. Closer to the main body of the Jewish community, we find the doctrine accepted by the Samaritans and Karaites and, more importantly, by Philo, the popular first-century philosopher of Alexandria. On the other hand, his younger contemporary Josephus bears witness to the Palestinian (halakhic) tradition. Aside from its textual warrant, this tradition is more authentic than the later tendency, "which, in addition, is not genuinely Jewish but must have originated in Alexandria under Egyptian-Greek influence."[7]

In the rabbinic tradition, then, abortion remains a noncapital crime at worst. But a curious factor further complicates the question. One more biblical text, this one in Genesis and hence "before Sinai" and part of the Laws of the Sons of Noah, served as the source for the teaching that feticide is indeed a capital crime—for non-Jews. Genesis 9:6 reads: "He who sheds the blood of man, through man [i.e., through the human court of law] shall his blood be shed." Since the "man, through man" (*shofekh dam ha' adam ba'adam*) can also be rendered "man, in man," the Talmud records the exposition of Rabbi Ishmael: "What is this 'man, in man'? It refers to the fetus in its mother's womb." Being in Genesis—without the qualifying balance of the Exodus (Sinaitic) passage—this verse made feticide a capital crime for non-Jews (those not heir to the covenant at Sinai) in Jewish law. Some hold this exposition to be more sociologically than textually inherent, voicing a reaction against abuses among the heathen. In view of rampant abortion and feticide, they claim, Rabbi Ishmael extracted from the Genesis text this judgment against the Romans.[8]

Regardless of rationale, the doctrine remains part of theoretical Jewish law, as Maimonides, for example, codifies it: "A 'Son of Noah' who killed a person, even a fetus in its mother's womb, is capitally liable. . . ." Therapeutic abortion is not, however, included in this Noahide prohibition; nor is an abortion during the first forty days, according to some. The implications of this anomaly—a different law for the Sons of Noah than for Israel —were addressed in a Responsum of the eighteenth century: "It is not to be supposed that the Torah would consider the embryo as a person [*nefesh*] for them [Sons of Noah] but not for us. The fetus is not a person for them either; the Torah was merely more severe in its practical ruling in their regard. Hence, therapeutic abortion would be permissible to them, too."[9]

If abortion is not murder in the rabbinic system, neither is it worse than murder. It is worse than murder in those religious systems concerned with "ensoulment" of the fetus. At a conference some time ago on the subject, I made bold to say that the discussion for the past several sessions of the conference was monumentally irrelevant. They had been debating the time of ensoulment—does the soul enter the fetus at conception, at the end of the first trimester, at birth? From the Jewish standpoint, this must be declared irrelevant. It's not when does the soul enter, it's what kind of a soul enters? Classic Christianity has been saying that a tainted soul enters the fetus which must be cleansed by baptism to save him or her from eternal perdition. In line with the doctrine of original sin, each individual soul inherits the taint of its primordial ancestors. When St. Fulgentius of the sixth century was asked when that stain attaches to the person, he replied that it begins with conception. Hence the concern with allowing the fetus to be brought to term so that it can be baptized; otherwise it is condemned to death in both worlds, making abortion clearly worse than murder. It must accordingly be said that when Catholics reputedly decide to "let the mother die" rather than allow an abortion, they are not at all being cruel, merely consistent with a logical concern. The mother has been presumably baptized as an infant; let her die and "go to her reward." But let the child be brought to term and baptized and saved from perdition. So sincere is this concern that theologians at the Sorbonne in the nineteenth century invented a baptismal syringe, wherewith to baptize a fetus in utero in the event of a spontaneous abortion, a miscarriage.[10]

But this is surely a concern that the Jewish community cannot share. Having no such concept of original sin, we recite daily in our prayers something that comes directly from the Talmud: "My God, the soul with which thou hast endowed me is pure." We inherit a pure soul, which becomes contaminated only by our own misdeeds. By that token, early abortion would send a fetus to heaven in a state of pristine purity! While the Talmud does discuss the time of ensoulment—is it when the child is conceived, or at the first trimester, at birth or, as one opinion has it, when the child first answers Amen?—but then dismisses the question as both unanswerable and irrelevant to the abortion question.[11]

Abortion then is neither murder nor worse than murder, nor an option when the alternative is death to the mother. Since the mother is not allowed to choose suicide, abortion in that extreme case becomes mandatory. This is the sense of the fundamental passage in the Talmud bearing on the subject. The Mishnah (*Oholot* 7,6) puts it this way:

"If a woman has [life-threatening] difficulty in childbirth, the embryo within her must be dismembered limb by limb [if necessary], because her life [*hayyeha*] takes precedence over its life [*hayyav*]. Once its head (or its greater part) has emerged, it may not be touched, for we may not set aside one life [*nefesh*] for another."

The justification for abortion then is that before the child emerges we do not yet have a *nefesh*. The life of the fetus is only potential, and that cannot compete with actual human life.

In a previous chapter, I related my experience at a conference in Rome. After presenting a Jewish view calling for abortion to avoid a threat to life, a Catholic woman physician challenged the point on the grounds of her own experience, where she had accepted the ruling of her priest against any abortion over the contrary advice of her doctor. But a priest present at the conference explained that while the Catholic faithful must obey the Church's teaching against abortion, a Jewish woman was equally duty-bound to follow the tenets of Jewish law. She must abide by the physician's determination that abortion is called for because her life is in danger, even if this later turns out to be mistaken. The priest correctly articulated the Jewish legal-moral position on the question.

Another such clarifying confrontation took place in New York City, when another Catholic woman rose to question the point of view. She began: "Don't you believe in the Bible?" Unsure of what she may have had in mind, I answered with a tentative yes. She said: "Well, the Bible says, 'Therefore, choose life.' Since abortion is the killing of life, how can you allow it?" "Because," I replied, "when you see 'choose life' in the Bible and when we see 'choose life' in the Bible, we are both seeing different things. From a Catholic standpoint, which is essentially other-worldly in orientation, you see 'life' as life in the next world. Otherwise, why would you ever allow the death of the mother? That, too, is taking life. Yet, you feel that the mother, having already been baptized, can 'choose life' in the next world. But when we see those words, we think of life in this world, and that's why we strive to save the mother, to save existing life. How do I know this? Because the Talmud gives the rationale for the principle that 'saving life sets aside all else in the Torah,' that the Sabbath and even Yom Kippur must be violated in order to protect or preserve life or health. The rationale is simple: 'Violate [for the patient] this Sabbath, so that he will be able to keep many Sabbaths.'[12] In other words, we want to 'choose life' here on earth, and a therapeutic abortion is therefore indicated, even mandated."

As cited at the outset, the Talmud considered basing the justification rather on the fact that the fetus is a *rodef*, an aggressor. Since the law of *rodef* allows us to kill the pursuer in order to save his intended victim, where we cannot stop him otherwise, the fetus may be defined in this way. But, says the Talmud, perhaps the mother is pursuing the child? The life-threatening impasse could be the result of a narrow cervix, or any physiological condition of the mother which makes continuation of the pregnancy a threat to her life. If the condition is the mother's, how is the child the pursuer? Rather, says the Talmud, "she is being pursued from Heaven." That is, the pursuit is an "act of God," desired or intended neither by mother or child. The argument is therefore inadmissible and, in any case, unnecessary; it's simply that the fetus is not yet a person with equal title to life.

Yet Maimonides, in his great summarizing Law Code, seems to retrieve the rejected argument. He formulates the talmudic law as follows:

"This, too, is a [negative] Commandment: Not to take pity on the life of a pursuer. Therefore the Sages ruled that when a woman has difficulty in giving birth, one dismembers the fetus in her womb—either with drugs or by surgery—because it is like a pursuer seeking to kill her. Once its head has emerged, it may not be touched, for we may not set aside one life for another; this is the natural course of the world."[13]

Since abortion is not murder, and Maimonides could not have ruled otherwise, the commentators on his Code explain that he made figurative use of the pursuer idea in order to buttress the justification for abortion when necessary. Hence his formulation *k'rodef*, that the fetus is "like a pursuer."

Illustrative of the difference, albeit technical, between murder and killing is the following report: Rabbi Issar Unterman, late Chief Rabbi of Israel, is firmly opposed to abortion except under extreme circumstances. He labels it "akin to murder," but preserves the distinction. He tells of a Jewish girl made pregnant by a German soldier during the First World War. She asked the soldier for support of the child to be born; he instead took her to a physician to abort. The physician, who was Jewish, declined to perform the abortion, insisting it was against his principles. The soldier then drew his gun and threatened the doctor: Either you abort or I will shoot you. Rabbi Unterman declared that, had he been asked the question by the doctor he would have told him to abort. If abortion were really murder, the doctor would have had to martyr himself, to lay down his life rather than comply. Much as I would like to call it murder, he said in effect, the clear sense of Jewish law is that it is not.

It might also be mentioned in this connection that Rabbi Joseph Rosin of

Rogatchov responded, in the early part of this century, to a query as to whether a man may divorce his wife because she brought about an abortion. His answer was "no": although abortion is "akin to homicide," it is not a real enough homicide or offense to make her divorcible against her will.[14]

Rabbi Unterman stood squarely in the tradition of Maimonides and, in fact, all rabbinic teaching on the subject of abortion can be said to align itself with either Maimonides, on the right, or with Rashi, on the left. The "rightist" approach begins with the assumption, formulated by Unterman, that abortion is "akin to murder" and therefore allowable only in cases of corresponding gravity, such as saving the life of the mother. The approach then builds *down* from that strict position to embrace a broader interpretation of life-saving situations. These include a threat to her health, for example, and perhaps a threat to her sanity in terms of suicidal possibilities, but excludes any lesser reasons.

The more "liberal" approach, based on Rashi's affirmation that the fetus is not a human person, is associated with another former Chief Rabbi of Israel, Ben Zion Uziel.[15] This approach assumes that no real prohibition against abortion exists and builds *up* from that ground to safeguard against indiscriminate or unjustified thwarting of potential life. This school of thought includes the example of Rabbi Yair Bachrach in the seventeenth century, whose classic Responsum saw no legal bar to abortion but would not permit it in the case before him.[16] The case was of a pregnancy conceived in adultery; the woman "in deep remorse," wanted to destroy the fruit of her sin. The Responsum concludes by refusing to sanction abortion, not on legal grounds, but on sociological ones, as a safeguard against further immorality.

Other authorities, such as Rabbi Jacob Emden, disagreed on this point, affirming the legal sanction of abortion for the woman's welfare, whether life or health, or even for avoidance of "great pain."

Maternal rather than fetal indications are the rule for both schools of thought. The rightist position certainly considers only the mother, but so does the leftist one. The latter school includes even the mother's less than life-and-death welfare, expressed in the words "great pain," and based on the principle that *tza'ara d'gufah kadim*. Rabbinic rulings on abortion, when collated and distilled, are thus amenable to the following generalization:

If a woman were to come before the rabbi and seek permission for an abortion by saying, "I had German measles, or I took Thalidomide during pregnancy, and the possibility is that the child will be born deformed," the rabbi would decline permission on those grounds. "How do you know," he might say, "that the child will be born deformed? Maybe not. And if so, how do you know that such a condition is worse for him than not being born? Why mix into 'the secrets of God'?" But if the same woman under the same circumstances came to the same rabbi and expressed the problem differently; if she said, "...the possibility is that the child will be born deformed, and that possibility is giving me extreme mental anguish," then the rabbi would rule otherwise. Now the fetal indication has become a maternal indication, and all the considerations for her welfare are now brought to bear. The fetus is unknown, future, potential, part of the "secrets of God"; the mother is known, present, human and seeking compassion.

One rabbinic authority, writing in Rumania in 1940, responded to the case of an epileptic mother who feared that her unborn child would also be epileptic.[17] He writes: "For fear of possible, remote danger to a future child that maybe, God forbid, he will know sickness—how can it occur to anyone to actively kill the fetus because of such a possible doubt? This seems to me very much like the laws of Lycurgus, King of Sparta, according to which every blemished child was to be put to death.... Permission for abortion is to be granted only because of mental anguish for the mother. But for fear of what might be the child's lot?—The secrets of God are not knowable."

He was, in fact, basing his decision on an explicit ruling in 1913 by Rabbi Mordecai Winkler of Hungary: "Mental-health risk has been definitely equated with physical-health risk. This woman, in danger of losing her mental health unless the pregnancy is interrupted, would therefore accordingly qualify."[18]

The emphasis on maternal as opposed to fetal indications caused a dilemma with regard to such tragic, but clearly fetal, afflictions as that of Tay-Sachs. Screening of prospective mates or parents is recommended; but after a pregnancy begins, may amniocentesis be performed in order to determine if the cells of the fetus have been affected? Having limited the warrant for abortion to maternal indications, and no risk to the mother's life or health exists even with the birth of a Tay-Sachs child, the answer would be negative. And since abortion is ruled out, amniocentesis itself would be halakhically proscribed as a gratuitous invasive assault, with its own attendant risks, upon the womb. The dilemma, however, is resolved by a perception on the part of the mother that this is really a maternal indication. The present knowledge that the child will deteriorate and die in infancy, although the birth itself will be safe for her, gives her genuine mental anguish now. The fetal indication has become a maternal one.

Alternatively, though the majority of halakhic positions are as described here, there are at least two eminent authorities who rule that some fetal indications, such as this one, are serious enough in themselves to warrant an abortion. Rabbi Saul Israeli of the Jerusalem Rabbinical Court and Rabbi Eliezer Waldenberg, an expert in medical ethics, have so ruled.[19]

The spectrum of Jewish positions on the matter of abortion, from right to left, stands in sharp contrast to its consensus on neonatal defectives. Here the attitude is starkly illiberal, making the Jewish tradition the real "right to life" affirmation. Another look at that passage from the Mishnah proves that all this concern for the welfare of the mother obtains prior to birth. From the moment of birth, the life of the infant is as inviolate as that of the mother. Its right to life is then absolute. Before birth, however, right to life is not the applicable concept; it is "right to be born." The right to be born is not absolute, but relative to the welfare of the mother. There is no right to be born any more than a right to be conceived. Use of the "right to life" slogan by antiabortion people is therefore essentially misleading.

But just as the Mishnah makes the fetus secondary to the mother before birth, so it rejects any distinction after birth. This negates another popular slogan, "quality of life." If quality of life were a factor, it would be absurd to say that the newborn babe is equal to its mother. The mother has her achievements and her interconnected dependencies; the infant has none of these yet. Still, we reject any considerations of relative quality; all existing life is equally precious; the operative slogan is rather "sanctity of life." From the moment of its birth, the life of the newborn is sacred, as indivisibly and undifferentially sacred as that of the mother. This is the true "right-to-life" position. Whereas "right to be born" is relative to the welfare of the mother, "right to life" is not relative to the mother's or anyone's welfare. Right to life means that *no person* need apologize for living, neither to parents, to physicians, to society, or to self.

The great pains this chapter takes to prove abortion warrantable under some circumstances should not obscure the fact that abortion retains its stigma and remains a last resort. Procreation is a positive mitzvah, and potential life has the sanctity of its potential. The Talmud, in fact, uses the dreaded word "murder" in a figurative, hyperbolic sense even in connection with not conceiving. Bachelors or the couple who decline to conceive are called "guilty of bloodshed" for their sin of omission. Procreation is a desideratum as well as a mitzvah, and casual abortion is accordingly abhorrent. There may be legal and moral sanction for abortion where necessary, but the attitude remains one of solemn hesitation in the presence of the sanctity of life and of a pronatalist respect for new life.

Accordingly, abortion for "population control" is repugnant to the Jewish mind. Abortion for economic reasons is also not admissible. Taking precaution by abortion or contraception against physical threat to the mother remains a mitzvah, but not so as to forestall financial difficulty. Material considerations or career concerns are simply improper in this connection, especially in view of the readiness of others to adopt or nurture. A degree of brutalization is scarcely avoidable in the destruction of even potential life or in the rejection of a precious gift of God. But when the reasons for considering abortion are nonetheless overwhelming, the right to do so remains hers after all.

In the course of the 1984 presidential campaign, Archbishop John O'Connor of New York made an impassioned plea for people of all religious and political persuasions to join in the struggle against abortion on demand and in support of reverence for life. The Jewish community applauds and shares in that battle, but also in the pluralistic concern for individual liberty. Some contemporary rabbis welcome the strong stand of antiabortion groups, and regard the leniencies of traditional Jewish law as either too subtle or too dangerous for broad consumption. Others see the right of choice as inherent in the Jewish treatment of the subject, and stress the noncapital nature of the offense. Either way, it is important that reverence for life be affirmed as a religious imperative, but that political candidates or parties not be allowed to equate abortion with murder and prochoice people with murderers or outlaws. Murder is a fundamental evil that no civilized society should tolerate, but abortion can be understood in more than one way; the right to it under circumstances consistent with conscience should not be compromised or unduly stigmatized.

· 10 ·

Right to Life—Neonatal and Terminal

If abortion, after all, concerns not the "right to life" but the "right to be born," it may at times be warranted in the name of a greater good, such as the welfare of the mother. There is, however, no greater good to which the life of a born child, a human person, may be subjugated. Right to life properly means that once a human being is born his title to life is inviolate, and its continuation need not consider the welfare of any other.

There were several "Baby Doe" situations that preceded the most recent, more celebrated ones. After an earlier case, the Kennedy Institute of Bioethics convened a conference on the subject. Parents of a child born with Down's syndrome had now been told that the baby suffered from other abnormalities that required surgery for correction. The parents reasoned that if they refused permission for surgery the child would die and they would not be burdened with a retardate. They refused permission, the child died—and there was a hue and cry throughout the land. Our medical ethics, it was claimed, as well as our hospital procedures, our legal ethics, and more, need radical revision, and hence that symposium.

At the symposium I was seated between two other speakers on the platform, with—as it happened—the one on my left espousing a "leftist" point of view and the speaker on my right representing a more rightist, conservative stance. The speaker on my right declared himself opposed to abortion under all circumstances, including that of a deformed fetus. Abortion is wrong, he said, even if the fetus is defective and, it goes without saying, the neonate should not be denied life if it is handicapped. The spokesman on my left insisted that not only is abortion indicated if the fetus is impaired, but—why limit ourselves to that? Why restrict this option to the prenatal stage only; why operate, so to speak, in the dark? Why not allow ourselves the first postnatal year to observe the child in the light of day and determine whether it is viable? Why not have the child on probation of sorts as we decide whether it should live or not?

I told the conference that not only was I seated in the middle between these two extremes, but that the Jewish position can be described as standing foursquare between them. I cited the two-part ruling of the Mishnah quoted in the previous chapter, with its apparent leniency in the first half and stringency in the second. The first allows abortion where necessary up until the moment of birth, at least theoretically: "The fetus is dismembered, limb by limb, for her [the mother's] life takes precedence over its life." This is "liberal," but its main point is that the fetus is secondary to the mother's welfare. The second part of the Mishnah places the life of the child on the same level as hers, because now we have two human persons: "Once the head has emerged (or, in the case of a breech birth, once half the body has emerged), it may not be touched, for we may not set aside one life for another."

Placing the two on the same level reflects the teaching that life is inviolable, despite the tendency to make distinctions on the basis of quality or other criteria. As said above, the slogan "quality of life" is inadmissible in these situations; it must yield to the preferred slogan, "sanctity of life." If relative quality were a consideration, surely the mother has more. She has husband or other children dependent upon her; she has her proven viability and her social interconnections. The newborn babe has none of these. Yet, no distinctions are allowable: Life is sacred, in undifferentiated preciousness. Similarly, if the state of the child's health is not up to par, its title to life is undiminished. Life is sacred and must be safeguarded against active homicide or passive neglect.

The Jewish community accordingly welcomed in principle the position taken by the Reagan Administration in intervening in Baby Doe cases. It claimed that a handicapped child has as much right to vigorous life-sustaining treatment, let alone to be saved from passive euthanasia, as does the healthy child. We applauded this act in the name of the principle of the sanctity of life, although we asked that either the government or private social agencies remove the bulk of the financial and emotional burden from the parents. As opposed to abortion, where government denial of right is wrongful interference in a matter of personal conscience, deprivation of the right to life from an existing human is a violation of an objective principle. In testimony before representatives of the administration on this point, I indicated that the principle of the sanctity of life is supreme above all other considerations. It is not up to the parents to make the decision, nor is it up to the physicians to make the determination on the basis of projected quality of life; it is not even up to the child to decide on suicide or not. It is only the objective principle that can "decide." The answer to the dramatic question "Whose life is it anyway?" is not the one implied by the sardonic "anyway" of the phrasing. Life is God's, and no subjective considerations can allow us to commit either suicide or homicide. An infant may lack quality of life, but we must tend it and are forbidden to end its life by commission or omission. If it sometimes seems a great pity to keep it alive, that is the price we must pay for seeking to uphold the principle. The alternative is unthinkable: It opens the door to arrogating to ourselves the right to murder, which is unacceptable either in the hands of a well-meaning physician or parent, or of a malevolent Nazi.

It must also be said that an unswerving affirmation of existing life leads to creative efforts to sustain and enhance it. Doctors at Hadassah Hospital in Israel have perfected a plastic-surgery technique for correcting the appearance of Down's syndrome children. Often their intelligence is but slightly lower than that of the rest of us, but the Mongoloid shape of their eyes betrays them. Peers and teachers then assume they are incapable of keeping up with others, and they are relegated to special classes; this becomes a self-fulfilling prophecy. Plastic surgery reduces the appearance factor, and thus the prejudice, and gives them a far better chance in life. Such medical advances are the direct result of the human postulate and position that life is precious and must be preserved and nurtured.

All of this holds equally true for the other end of life or for mortally ill patients at any age. Nothing may be done to hasten death even by a moment, for this too is murder.

The Talmud outlines the procedure to be followed immediately after death. The eyes, if open, must be closed; the hands and feet must be brought together. To carry out any of these or other procedures while life is ebbing, however, is thereby to hasten death. The soul is likened to the flame on a candle; to touch a flickering candle is to put out the flame prematurely. Even to hasten death by psychological means is forbidden; hence the deathbed confessional, as indicated above, is couched in the conditional mode. Rather than abandon the will to live by stating "I am about to die," the patient asks for continued life; only if this cannot be does he confess his sins and ask for a share in the World to Come.

Neither active nor passive hastening of death is permitted. The patient has no "autonomy," and life is not "his" to take, certainly not anyone else's to take. Withdrawal of artificial support systems is, in principle, no different from withdrawal of food from a starving person. Under what circumstances, then, may one "pull the plug"?

A striking narrative in the Talmud (*Avodah Zarah* 18a) implicitly offers some guidance on this subject. The passage has to do with the martyr's death of Rabbi Hanina ben Teradyon, along with the deaths of several other rabbis who were executed by the Romans for the sin of teaching Torah. The Romans had forbidden the teaching of Torah on penalty of death, but the rabbis heroically defied the ban. They cited the parable of the fox, who shrewdly seeks to entice the fish out of the water by pointing to some danger to them in the water. The fish reply that if their life is in danger in the water, how much more is it in danger out of the water. The rabbis similarly reasoned that if their lives are threatened when they teach Torah, they are no less in danger if they cease the study of Torah, "for it is our life and the length of our days."

Rabbi Akiva, incidentally, was put to death in a tortuous way by the Romans for violating the ban. He was wrapped in a scroll of the Torah and set on fire. He declared himself fortunate: "All my life I have tried to fulfill 'Love the Lord thy God with all thy heart and all thy soul and all thy might.' Only now can I love God with all my soul [life]." Also parenthetically, it was talmudic sages who "coined" the word euthanasia in Hebrew long before the Greek roots were used by Sir Thomas More to form the compound term. Even the convicted criminal, Rabbi Nahman taught, deserves compassion. If he must be executed, give him a narcotic so he will not suffer pain as he dies. This is in fulfillment of "Love thy neighbor as thyself," which includes, he taught, "choose for him a good death [*mitah yafah*, literally *eu-thanatos*, a good death]."[1]

In the case of Rabbi Hanina ben Teradyon, the Romans placed him in the fire for execution but covered his chest with woolen sponges drenched in water. This was to keep him alive longer while the fires burned and thus to prolong his agony. His disciples pleaded with him to overcome this evil device by opening his mouth wide so that he might be asphyxiated by the smoke, die more quickly and be spared the pain. He refused, says the Talmud, on the grounds that that would constitute suicide. "Only He Who gave life can take it away; I may not do it myself," he replied to his disciples in this incredible conversation. "Well, then," the executioner himself, who took pity on him, offered, "let me remove these moistened sponges from around your heart." That, he answered, is permissible. In the first case, the suggestion was one of hastening death by one's own action. That he could not allow. In the second, it was a case of removing an impediment, artificially supplied, that delayed the expected process of dying. Removing a hindrance to natural death is permitted. The executioner did so, and Rabbi Hanina's agony ended. When the executioner himself died, the Talmud reports, he "went straight to heaven" for this act of exquisite mercy, implying, of course, that the act was not only permissible but meritorious. We are even told that Rabbi Judah the Prince spoke enviously of him. Some of us, he said, strive throughout our lifetimes to earn a place in the World to Come, but some earn their place there in a single moment of great righteousness!

A clear distinction is thus implied between the deliberate termination of life and the removal of means that artificially prolong the process of death. Jewish law codes subsequently make the teaching explicit: To "remove hindrances" to the "soul's departure" is permitted and even mandated.[2] While physicians, then, may not disconnect life-support systems where they shorten life thereby, they may do so to shorten the death process. Since, however, we "begin dying the moment we are born" and, more to the point, it is difficult to tell the difference between shortening life and death, the principle is a moral one more than a practical one. At the outset, the physician should connect the support systems of respiration or circulation; he should not decline to do so on the grounds that this may be prolonging death. He must give the patient every chance for life. Having connected the systems conditionally, however, he may remove them if he then determines that their function was not prolongation of life but of death. This provisional procedure at least precludes the active termination of systems for any other reason.

Even passive euthanasia is forbidden in principle. After all, what difference can be drawn between withholding artificial support systems and withholding food or drink from one who would otherwise passively starve to death? Insulin is artificial food, and to withhold it from the diabetic is to cause his death; no difference applies either because the food is artificial or the withholding is passive. And the injunction against suicide/homicide is not rendered inapplicable because of the existence of pain or poor quality of life.

Yet, passive euthanasia may be permitted where active is not, in special cases of the terminally ill. The patient really has no "autonomy" to choose the cessation of natural or artificial life support. But he does have the choice to refuse further active treatment, such as surgery, when the risk-benefit ratio is not in his favor. Cardiopulminary resuscitation is in itself a traumatic assault, and some procedures to overcome a developing crisis are in themselves a risk. The patient's implied autonomy to refuse hazardous or counterproductive treatment may be a determining factor in opting for palliative rather than curative therapy.

Some contemporary rabbinic authorities go a bit further. Conscious of the halakhic dialectic between two serious considerations—the infinite preciousness of life, on the one hand, and both the concern with avoidance of unnecessary pain and the express mandate to remove hindrances to the dying process, on the other—some have written to permit passive cessation of efforts in specific cases. One eminent authority, who would not allow the withholding of natural means of subsistence such as food and water for a painfully terminal patient, would permit the cessation of medical treatment.[3] Another sanctioned the decision to refrain from providing insulin to a diabetic who also suffered from a severely painful cancer.

In the human situation before us, the principles struggle for assertion. Having affirmed our bias for life, our reverence for life's sanctity in spite of pain and infirmity, and our compelling mandate to heal, we seek the right resolution. The dialectic between the two moral thrusts, that of the preciousness of life and the imperative to extend mercy to our fellow-man, even to the convicted criminal, allows the application of the practical principle of *shev v'al ta'aseh*, "sit back and take no action," that is, let nature take its course. In such cases, "do not resuscitate" would be the proper procedure.

· 11 ·

Aging, Death, and Afterlife

"Until Jacob there was no sickness," says the Talmud (*Bava Metzia* 87a). It was a favor to him, and to everyone else, because it prepares one for death in a practical way. It enables one to "put his affairs in order," as the text implies: "It was told to Joseph, behold your father is sick; and he brought his two sons with him" (Gen. 48:1). Similarly, the Talmud tells us, "Until Abraham there was no old age." It was a favor to him and to the rest of us.

Length of days is the promise held out in return for observance of the laws of the Torah; length of days is the anticipated blessing. "To life," and "till 120 years" are mutual salutations, the latter probably based on the reference in Genesis 6:3 or on the fact that such was the lifespan of Moses. Yet, "our days are but seventy years and, by strength, eighty years," says the Psalmist (90:10). Whether the lifespan is less or more than that, the prayer is for a *good* old age, *seivah tovah* (Gen. 15:15).

Old age that is not so good is described classically in Ecclesiastes 12. There the infirmities of advanced age are put in striking images, and the Talmud elaborates on the meaning of the verses in terms of the human condition. In the sixteenth and seventeenth centuries, John Smith and others explained the words of Ecclesiastes 12 in medical terms, while Arthur Schopenhauer in the nineteenth century wrote that one has to reach the age of seventy to appreciate the "vanity of vanities, all is vanity" of that biblical book.

Respect for the aged is preeminent in the ethical code of Leviticus (19:32), and disrespect for one's elders is the sign of a corrupt generation in Isaiah (3:5). The Sanhedrin is made up of elders, whose greater experience equals greater wisdom, and leaders and sages are called elders. Yet, the provision for the make-up of the Sanhedrin also calls for the exclusion of the very old, the difference between the two not exactly defined. For it is not chronological age but the condition of one's faculties that makes the difference, and a cogent statement of the Talmud accords with the findings of modern science. Barring the intrusion of ill health, the powers of the mind do indeed increase with age and experience, providing they have not been neglected. "Disciples of the wise increase in mental acuity as they age; the empty-headed increase in mental deficiency as they age" (*Shabbat* 152b). Recent scientific tests point to the truth that "if you don't use it, you lose it"; that the one who continues in active use of the mind remains or grows in mental sharpness.[1] Without a decline in physical health, only self-fulfilling prophecies contribute to the myth that older people are somehow deficient in either memory or sharpness of mind.

Age must be respected because of its presumed greater wisdom, but even more so because of greater infirmities. Proper treatment of and care for the aged is fundamental to the ethical code, and the individual mitzvah has, historically, been fulfilled both at home within the family circle and in institutions, known as *Moshav Zekenim*. The latter attend to routine needs, but the human ones come from personal attention by family in or out of institutions.

In a sense, the teaching that age must be respected can derive from another human value, other than either the greater wisdom of the aged or their greater infirmity, calling upon us ethically for higher regard. One of my hospital experiences included the following scenario: The patient reported some excitement in the corridors the night before. The hospital has an airway unit, to relieve breathing obstruction, manned by an airway-unit team. A patient who feels a choking sensation pushes a panic button and the team rushes in with the unit to relieve the problem. The patient that night was a ninety-year-old woman, and so the team, a group of interns, was overheard complaining in the corridors. "Imagine," they said, "disturbing our sleep at night for a ninety-year-old woman!" The chief of interns heard it, too, and called them together for a reprimand: "A woman that age," he told them, "has as much right to her life, and to our vigorous efforts to preserve that life, as someone nine or nineteen. Let me not hear you making such wrong judgments again."

From the Judaic point of view, one can add that she may have even more of a right to life. If, among other things, the human soul is the repository of one's feelings, experiences, memories and the like, then the older the person the greater the capacity of the soul. The opposite point of view judges a person by his productivity, by what or how much he or she can produce and contribute to economic or social life. But that materialistic valuation, we are taught, must be avoided in favor of a spiritual yardstick that judges one for what he is rather than for what he does. The elders may or may not have more wisdom, but they do have unique quality from this viewpoint.

The procedure at the moment of death is specified in the Talmud and legal tradition. If the eyes remain open, they are to be closed, the hands and feet brought together. The *chevra kadisha*, the "holy society" organized for this purpose, attends to *taharah*, the cleansing of the body, and the family prepares for immediate burial.

Immediate burial is considered an expression of respect for the sanctity of the body, and burial as opposed to cremation or other alternatives is part of the procedure mandated by the Torah. If even for the convicted and executed criminal the Bible commands ". . . his body shall not remain overnight [hanging] on the tree, but you shall certainly bury him on that day . . ." (Deut. 21:23), then the rest of us, we may infer, are also to be given that respect. Funerals accordingly take place as soon as possible after death, consistent with the principle of respect for the deceased. This includes enabling the relatives to be present as soon as physically possible, but not merely as soon as convenient. It is interesting to note that, whereas criteria for a definition of the moment of death have been refined, the Jewish practice of immediate burial was, in the past, the target of scorn. Civil authorities recommended a waiting period of seventy-two hours following clinical signs of death before permitting burial. Rabbi Moses Mendelsohn, a leading figure in the nineteenth-century Enlightenment, had to deal with Napoleon and his representatives on this matter.

Since burial, as opposed to its alternatives, is mandated by the Torah, it is not subject to the wishes of either deceased or bereaved. Other mourning procedures, the week of *shivah*, the reciting of Kaddish, the eulogy, etc., fall into the category of *yekara d'shakhva*, honor of the deceased, or *y'kara d'hayei*, honor of the living. Theoretically, the deceased can have ordered that mourning rites for his honor, such as Kaddish, be waived; he cannot ask that burial be avoided in favor of, say, cremation, for that violates the biblical injunction independent of one's wishes. Some more liberal interpreters see the biblical command as requiring attention of any kind, namely that the body not be abandoned, but find cremation objectionable for other reasons. Recent rabbinic decisions have allowed cremated remains, after the fact, to be interred in Jewish cemeteries provided they are placed in a coffin for burial.

The importance of attention to burial is reflected in another concept, that of *met mitzvah*. It is a mitzvah not only to escort the dead to their resting place along with the family of mourners, but a special mitzvah to see to the burial of one who dies without family or friends to attend to him. This is underscored by the provision that even a *kohen*, nay even the high priest himself, should occupy himself with the burial of the friendless or unclaimed body. A *kohen* is not permitted to come in contact with the dead; but when confronted with an unburied corpse, even the high priest must defile himself and attend to this *met mitzvah*.

With burial completed, the mourners return to their homes to begin the period of *shivah* and other mourning rites. The principle of "Do not mourn overmuch" is expressed by the fact that *shivah*, which means "seven" is observed for six days and a fraction of the seventh; that *sh'loshim*, the thirty-day period of lesser mourning, extends for twenty-nine days and a fraction; and even the year-long mourning, of a still lesser degree, lasts for eleven months with only a fraction of the last day of the eleventh month. Then the *Yahrzeit*, the anniversary of the death, is observed thereafter. The idea is to do less rather than too much mourning; enough for adequate expression of grief but not an irreverent dwelling on self-pity. Actually, the mourning period for all relatives was originally the thirty-day period only, but was extended in the case of parents for a year. Obviously, this is for respect more than for grief. The grief one feels at the loss of a child is profound; and the Talmud tells us that "when a man dies, he dies to his wife; when a woman dies, she dies to her husband"—the grief at the loss of a spouse is more profound and bereaving than the loss of another relative. The death of a child, spouse or sibling calls for a mourning period of only thirty days. But the death of parents, who may no longer figure so prominently in our lives as we look horizontally to wife or husband or downward to our children and the future—for them the Tradition calls for an extended period of mourning for a year, to express the respect owed to them but sometimes forgotten in the horizontal or other involvements.

Life is indeed precious, Judaism is a this-worldly faith, we are bidden to set aside the Torah to avoid a threat to life or health—and yet, belief in the afterlife is a strong reality. "This world is an antechamber leading into the main room. Prepare yourself in the antechamber to enter the main room," we are taught in the mishnaic tractate *Ethics of the Fathers*.

Unlike what is to be found in the works of Dante, we are offered no topographical description of the next world, and at times concepts of the World to Come blend with visions of Messianic days on this earth. But the Talmud distinguishes clearly: "The difference between the Messianic days and this world is only the removal of oppression." That is, the Messiah will bring this-worldly relief from oppression and affliction. Significant in terms of our present theme is the popular tradition that the Messiah, when he comes, will heal the incurably lame and handicapped. The great hope is for redemption from both social and physical ills.

But two more otherworldly concepts need clarification. The Sabbath prayerbook has a passage in which all three are referred to: the days of the Messiah, the World to Come, and the Resurrection. To Maimonides, the World to Come describes a spiritual immortality. The physical resurrection will take place, too, because the doctrine includes it; but it will be a temporary miracle, soon to give way to the more logical immortal life of the soul without the body. More logical? The late Professor Morris Raphael Cohen used to claim that physical resurrection is the more logical. Never having seen a disembodied soul, he said, I cannot conceive of such a thing; but having seen body and soul together—of that I can conceive, as David Hume pointed out in another context. The more current version of this position is the claim that the mind needs the brain. How is survival of the mind possible when the brain grows senile or when the brain deteriorates completely in death? To which the response is usually given that in the present arrangement the mind needs the physical brain, just as a space traveler needs his spacesuit when on the moon but can discard it when back on earth. The mind and soul are of God and transcend the body and its limitations.

In the medieval Jewish philosophic understanding, heaven and hell may be understood more as a state of being than a location. When the soul is freed from its earthly frame, and only then, it can experience association with God, the Soul of the world. The meaning, then, of "For no man can see me and live" (Ex. 33:20) is not to prohibit or deny this possibility, but to make it possible only for afterlife, only for when the "man" does no longer "live" in the constraining body. In the body he can see only what human sense receptors allow him to see; freed of the body he can perceive what the soul can perceive. If, now, the soul had become contaminated by sin while with the body, it is estranged or distanced from God, and this is hell. If it had remained pure, it enjoys the bliss of unhampered association with God, and this is heaven or paradise.

The Midrash responds to doubt about the afterlife with a striking story of twins conversing in their mother's womb.[2] The first child to be is unhappy with his predicament in the dark and crowded room. His sibling seeks to comfort him: "Don't feel so bad about your life here. It's only temporary. Soon you will be born, which means, soon you will leave this dark existence and break forth into a bright and expansive world, with all kinds of delights to interest you." But it didn't help much; the first remained skeptical. "That's a lot of nonsense that some would have us believe," he said. "There is really nothing at all out there after this."

The hereafter is there but is not the focus of our attention or our efforts. Emphasis on otherworldly directedness is not the norm, but it has some illustrious proponents. Rabbi Moses Hayyim Luzzatto was a celebrated mystic and moralist of eighteenth-century Italy. His widely studied *Path of the Upright* sees this world as a means to the next, that man is here only, by diligent performance of the mitzvot, to earn his place there. As an example of its influence, it is told that a devout student in a European Yeshivah had been immersing himself in the study of Luzzatto's work, only to exclaim afterward: "All very true, but this world is *also* a world." The paradox is to be found once again in the *Ethics of the Fathers* (4:17): "Better one hour of repentance and good deeds in this world than the whole life of the World to Come. But better is one hour of spiritual bliss in the World to Come than the whole life of this world."

· 12 ·

Moment of Death, Transplantation, and Autopsy

Concern with the preciousness of every moment of life, on the one hand, and with attending to burial without delay, on the other, impels us to fix with some precision the moment of death. The third reason is more practical: to be able to save the life of one in need of a transplanted organ without hastening the death of the donor or diminishing the usefulness of the donated organ.

Criteria for determining death in Jewish law have their origin in the context of a talmudic discussion, once again, of Sabbath laws. The Mishnah (*Yoma* 85a) provides: If one comes across a collapsed structure on the Sabbath, he may remove the debris only if there is a chance of saving the life of one felled by the collapse and buried beneath it. If he does find a person there, he may remove enough debris to determine whether he's still alive; if he's not, he may not continue until after the Sabbath. How can one tell if the person is still alive? "Examine him at the nostrils," says the Mishnah. If you detect breathing at the nostrils, then you know he's alive and you may proceed. Alternatively, "Examine him at the heart." The two provisions together give us the indicia of death that prevailed until modern times, namely respiration and heartbeat. These are the external evidences of *yetziat neshamah*, the soul's departure, which is not subject to empirical observation.

Between the two, examination at the nostrils is more definitive, especially when heartbeat could not so easily be detected without a stethoscope. But Rabbi Zevi Ashkenazi (eighteenth century) ruled that cardiac activity is the crucial criterion, with respiration only an indicator of the presence of heartbeat.[1] Moreover, Rabbi Moses Sofer (nineteenth century) declared that a person may not be pronounced dead unless he "lies as still as an inan-

103

imate stone and there is no pulse [heartbeat] whatsoever."[2] This is in keeping with Rashi's comment on the talmudic passage that these criteria presuppose that the person is "like a corpse that does not move its limbs," which means that if he does move, the other two criteria cannot make him dead.

Nor does the use of an artificial respirator deprive a person of his aliveness, because his heart beats in an entirely normal and spontaneous manner. The respirator merely helps the breathing process. Hence, such a patient must be considered alive even if comatose. The heart-lung machine, on the other hand, does the work of a heart, too, but can sustain life only for a very short period, such as during open-heart surgery. Here, too, the patient with admittedly artificial supports must be declared alive. Accordingly, criteria of death must be stated as the *irreversible* cessation of respiration and cardiac activity.

In the current effort to make healthy organs available for transplant, and to reduce the financial and emotional burden of sustaining the lives of incurable patients, the criterion of "brain death" has been introduced. In October of 1984, the New York State Court of Appeals ruled that so-called brain-dead patients may be legally considered dead. The Court stated: "Ordinarily, death will be determined according to the traditional criteria of irreversible cardiorespiratory repose. When, however, the respiratory and circulatory functions are maintained by mechanical means, their significance as signs of life is at best ambiguous." Under such circumstances, the court acknowledged that death may be said to have occurred "when the entire brain's function has irreversibly ceased."

The brain-death criterion does have precedent, and acceptability, in Jewish law, but only if that phrase, "the entire brain's function," is included in the definition. The noted formulation of the Ad Hoc Committee of the Harvard Medical School, defining brain death as unresponsiveness to painful stimuli and a flat electroencephalogram, etc., was endorsed by the American Medical Association, the American Bar Association, and the President's Commission for the Study of Ethical Problems in Medicine. The latter's recommendation specified "irreversible cessation of all functions of the entire brain, including the brain stem."

Jewish law requires that specification, for a criterion of death based on higher cerebral or cortical cessation alone—without extending it to the vegetative functions of the vital centers of the brain stem—is morally unacceptable. And, for this criterion, there is talmudic precedent in the situation of decapitation. Even if there is convulsive reflex movement after decapitation, the Mishnah implies, there is still obvious evidence of death.

Modern rabbinic authorities subsume total brain-stem death under the category of decapitation. The heart may still be beating but, with a brain stem irreversibly gone, the patient is dead and his functioning heart can conceivably be used as a transplant to save the life of another.

In the case of heart transplantation, where timing is exquisitely delicate, two separate medical teams are especially necessary. The donor team would assure that the donor is in fact dead; to hasten his death by one second is to be guilty of murder. Without conflict of interest, then, the donee team can assure that the heart is sound and see to its proper implantation in the body of the recipient. In the case of other organs, such as liver, kidney, or cornea, their usefulness remains intact for a longer period.

Of course, the problem of timing is irrelevant where the organ is not taken from a human donor. An artificial heart, for example, eliminates the concerns connected with determination of the donor's death, and the heart of a baboon shifts the ethical focus to man's relation to the animal world. Judaism has much to say about the latter, offering a position that, on the one hand, asserts man's supremacy over the beast and that the animal kingdom is at the service of mankind and, on the other hand, has a remarkable set of rules against cruelty to animals. The phrase is *tza'ar ba'alei hayyim*, "prevention of pain to living creatures," and is reflected in many of the biblical commandments, such as against harnessing two animals of different strengths together for plowing, against muzzling the ox when it plows among the corn, and many other rules. The principle is seen in the dietary laws, where the process of slaughter must be painless, and in the historic abhorrence by Jews of hunting as a sport. If we are to partake of animal flesh or animal hide for the quality of our life, this does not make it permissible to cause unnecessary pain or death to animals. Ironically, kosher slaughter has come under criticism, in spite of this great moral contribution to civilization, because of another dietary concern. That is, in addition to painless slaughter, kosher laws require that the blood be drained as thoroughly as possible, since the blood may not be eaten.

Eating blood has negative associations with bloodthirstiness; the Bible says, "But the blood ye may not eat, for the blood is the life" (Deut. 12:23). To some this was taken to forbid transfusions; to the Jewish community transfusions were never an issue, but the eating of blood is very much an issue. Hence the slaughter of animals also required that they not be stunned first by a blow on the head, which would have congealed the blood or inhibited its free flow. The swiftness of razor-sharp slaughter avoided both cruelty to animals and consumption of residual blood.

Fundamental to the Judaic tradition here is the law that a limb torn from a live animal may not be eaten, that an animal may never be boiled while still alive, and other teachings that stress that animals, though in the service of man, may not be mistreated. Research on laboratory animals, if done purposively and without unnecessary pain, may be pursued to enhance the life of mankind. In the absence of human organs, then, the heart of a baboon may theoretically be used to save the life of a human infant. The example of blood, however, with its psychological association with the essence of life, may apply here as well. Implantation of an animal heart, as opposed to other animal organs, continues to be resisted on grounds that the heart is too closely associated with the essence of a person. Otherwise, the proper use of animal organs, properly obtained, is in accordance with Jewish legal standards.

Returning to the subject of transplants from human donors, it must be said that, even before the matter of timing is resolved, there is a prior question to be settled. Jewish law requires procedures of respect for the dead, of treating the body with a sanctity that remains with the body even after the soul's departure. This has implications for autopsy, but also for transplants. The principle is known as *nivvul ha-met*, that is, not to desecrate or mistreat the body. With regard to transplantation, the problem is solved easily: If the life of another can be saved, the interdiction against *nivvul ha-met* should certainly be set aside, just as other prohibitions are set aside when a life is at stake. The late Rabbi Issar Unterman, Chief Rabbi of Israel, accordingly ruled that a heart transplant under the right conditions is no less than a mitzvah; if the donor has definitely died and the heart can save a life, there is neither hastening of death nor desecration of the dead, only mitzvah.

Probably a more significant contribution to rabbinic legislation in this area is his extension of the concept to corneal transplants. After all, a person's life is not threatened by failure to receive a good cornea; how can we set aside the prohibition of desecrating the body of the donor? Because, Rabbi Unterman declared, saving eyesight is as important as saving life; surely it's important enough to set aside this consideration.[3]

But may it now be set aside to allow for an autopsy? The question has an interesting history, with a resolution that accommodates two important values. The one is to preserve the sanctity of the person's body, the other is to allow for the saving of life, directly or indirectly. Involved also are considerations of protecting the unprotected, of safeguarding the body of a person who can no longer fend for himself. Emotions run high in discussing the issue, but a modus vivendi is close at hand.

The classic ruling on the subject was given in the eighteenth century by Rabbi Ezekiel Landau of Prague.[4] The question addressed to him came from London, then a center for the study of anatomy. A man suffering from stones in his bladder died in unsuccessful surgery. The doctors wanted an autopsy in order to learn what went wrong and to do better the next time. The local rabbinic scholars had been divided on the issue: Some argued that the good that will accrue to society is ultimately an honor rather than dishonor to the deceased; others pointed to a passage in the Talmud against disinterment to solve a forensic question, on grounds of *nivvul ha-met*. Rabbi Landau responded by taking for granted that this prohibition is set aside to save life, but stipulated that there be a direct connection. Otherwise this person's body is being desecrated for some merely possible ultimate benefit. The words he used, the two crucial ones to be quoted again and again, were *holeh lefaneinu*, "a patient at hand." If there is a patient now with us in need of the information to save his life, then the autopsy is directly lifesaving, otherwise not. The doctor may violate the Sabbath to save life; he may not do so to prepare medicines that he may someday need.

Subsequent rabbinic authorities have carried the ruling to its logical conclusion in the light of modern technology. Because the results of an autopsy in London can be telegraphed or electronically transmitted to a hospital in New York, Jerusalem or Vienna, the whole world is now "at hand" or "before us." We are all, in Marshall McLuhan's phrase, part of a "global village" with the results in one place available to, and needed by, people everywhere. But this still precludes the performance of post-mortem operations to save no one's life, merely to add to the store of medical knowledge or to assist in training, and imposes the burden of demonstrating that there is a discernible connection between the dispensation and the good it will do. It also helps safeguard other aspects of the dispensation, such as that the parts removed for autopsy be returned to the body for burial, rather than disposed of down the drain. In 1954, Hadassah Hospital and Chief Rabbi Isaac Herzog came to terms in a concordat that allowed for autopsies to (a) save lives directly with the medical information garnered, (b) to save a life forensically, such as when the information will affect a defendant on trial, and (c) to save lives in the family when a hereditary condition is involved.

The struggle for and against post-mortem investigation continues, with arguments marshaled on both sides. Some center their debate on the question of whether autopsies are indeed as necessary as they used to be. Penicillin, heart surgery, polio vaccination—the knowledge for these advances didn't even come from autopsies; for other conditions, most of the relevant knowledge has already been gathered. In a number of cases, peritoneoscopy, a procedure that requires no incision on the body, or needle biopsy, which involves no invasive assault on the body, can yield the needed information. On the other side, Alzheimer's disease, and even AIDS, challenge us urgently to find cause, direction and cure of the disease. All scientific means of inquiry should be pressed into service without undue delay. The impasse involves, as well, organ donations and organ banks. The Rabbinate of Israel, while ready to permit the grafting of skin, for example, from a cadaver to a live victim of burns, has stated its opposition to storage of skin or organs against time of need. To do so is to desecrate the dead; but not to do so until need, as in a recent harrowing instance, is to hinder the speed and effectiveness of the grafting. A formula is being devised to respect both principles—preserving the dignity of the deceased and serving the vital health needs of the living—as much as conscience and practicality will allow.

These smaller battles are all part of the overall struggle, the effort to strike a balance between equal but conflicting values. The effort, in turn, is in the service of the goal of honoring God by holding life sacred, to be preserved and enhanced in wholesomeness of body and spirit.

Notes

Chapter 1/The Mandate to Heal

1. Maimonides, *Mishneh Torah, Deot* 3:3.
2. *Midrash Temurah*, in J. D. Eisenstein, *Otzar Midrashim*, vol. II, pp. 580–81.
3. Maimonides, Commentary on the Mishnah, *Nedarim* 4:4.
4. I. M. Rabbinowitz, *Rabbi Jacob Israel of Pzhsysha* (Piotrkow, 1932), pp. 59–60.
5. *Eikhah Rabbati* 6; Jeru. *Hagigah I,7*.
6. Genesis Rabbah 9:5.
7. *Shabbat* 31b, Mishnah.
8. *Yevamot* 12b and parallels.

Chapter 2/"Set Aside the Torah" to Protect Life and Health

1. I Maccabees 2:31–38, 40–41; Mark 2:27.
2. *Berakhot* 32b. See Maharsha, ad loc.
3. *Bava Kamma* 15b.
4. Responsa *Binyan Tziyyon* (Altona, 1868), no. 137.
5. Louis Ginzberg, *Students, Scholars and Saints* (Philadelphia: Jewish Publication Society, 1928), p. 192.

Chapter 3/Prayer and Concern for the Ill

1. Mishnah *Avot* 3:19.
2. *Sanhedrin* 101a; Mekhilta to Exodus 16:26.
3. *Pesahim* 64b; *Avodah Zarah* 18a.
4. *Ketubot* 104a.
5. *Nedarim* 39b.
6. *Kitzur Shulhan Arukh* 193:1–5.

Chapter 4/Judaism and Health

1. *HaTalmud V'Hokhmat HaRefuah* (Berlin, 1928), pp. 16–20.
2. See Fred Rosner, *Medicine in the Bible and Talmud* (New York: Ktav, 1977), p. 16.

3. Responsa *Teshuvah MeAhavah*, vol. III, *Yoreh Deah*, no. 336.
4. *Shulhan Arukh Yoreh Deah* 249:16; 255:2.
5. *Tosafot, Moed Katan* 11a; *Shulhan Arukh Orah Hayyim* 173; and *Magen Avraham* thereto.
6. Joshua Trachtenberg, *Jewish Magic and Superstition* (New York: Columbia University Press, 1939, 1961), passim.
7. See Eugene Cohen, *Guide to Ritual Circumcision and Redemption of the First-Born Son* (New York: Ktav, 1984), pp. 134–40.
8. Responsa *Beit Yisrael* (Buenos Aires, 1954), no. 152.
9. *The Jerusalem Post*, International Edition, December 1, 1984, p. 18.

Chapter 5/Jews and Medicine

1. For this chapter see Harry Friedenwald, *Jews and Medicine and Jewish Luminaries in Medical History*, 3 vols., rev. ed. (New York: Ktav, 1967).
2. David Rosner, *A Once Charitable Enterprise: Hospitals and Health Care in Brooklyn and New York, 1855–1915* (New York: Cambridge University Press, 1982).
3. *Encyclopedia Judaica*, vol. XI, pp. 1185–1204.

Chapter 6/Mental as well as Physical Health

1. Nahmanides, *Torat HaAdam*.
2. Israel Meir Mizrahi, Responsa *Pri HaAretz* (Jerusalem, 1899), *Yoreh Deah*, no. 2.
3. Responsa *Levushei Mordekhai, Hoshen Mishpat*, no. 39.
4. E.g., Responsa *Minhat Yitzhak*, vol. I, no. 115; Responsa *Igg'rot Mosheh, Even HaEzer*, no. 65.
5. David M. Feldman and Fred Rosner, eds., *Compendium on Medical Ethics* (New York: Federation of Jewish Philanthropies, 1984), pp. 75–78.
6. See addendum to the work *Melekhet Heresh* by Yehezkel Hefetz (Vilna, 1875).
7. See Simchah Bunim Sofer, Responsa *Shevet Sofer, Even HaEzer*, no. 21.
8. Text of the *k'tubbah* is suggested in, e.g., Resp. *Ginnat V'radim* (*Even HaEzer* 1:13) of Rabbi Abraham ben Mordecai (Constantinople, 1717).
9. Responsa *Minhat Yitzhak*, vol. I, no. 37, and vol. II, no. 17.

Chapter 7/Marriage and Marital Relations

1. Derrick Sherwin Bailey, *Sexual Relations in Christian Thought* (New York: Harper and Bros., 1959). See also David M. Feldman, *Birth Control in Jewish Law* (New York: New York University Press, 1968), pp. 81–99 (published in paperback with same pagination, as *Marital Relations, Contraception and Abortion in Jewish Law* [New York: Schocken Books, 1974]). Henceforth referred to as BCJL.
2. *Ketubbot* 61b, 62b; *Yad, Ishut* 14,2; *Shulhan Arukh Even HaEzer* 76,5.
3. *Ketubbot* 56a; *Yad, Ishut* 12,7; BCJL, pp. 63–65.
4. John T. Noonan, Jr., *Contraception: A History of Its Treatment by the Catholic Theologians and Canonists* (Cambridge, Mass.: Harvard University Press, 1965), pp. 97, 98, 528. For Calvin, see his *Commentarius in Genesium*, ad loc.

5. Nathan Drazin, *Marriage Made in Heaven* (New York: Abelard-Schuman, 1958), p. 59.
6. Rabbi Hayyim Sofer, Responsa *Mahaneh Hayyim* (Pressburg, 1862), no. 53.
7. *Yevamot* 62b, *Pesahim* 72b; *Shulhan Arukh Orah Hayyim* 240,1.
8. H. E. Sigerest, *A History of Medicine* (New York: Oxford University Press, 1951), pp. 62–64.
9. Responsa *Hatam Sofer, Even HaEzer*, no. 20.
10. *Yevamot* 65b, *Perek HaShalom*, addendum to *Massekhet Derekh Eretz Zuta; BCJL*, pp. 43–45.
11. Jacob Milgrom, "The Case of the Suspected Adulteress," in *The Creation of Sacred Literature*, ed. R. F. Friedman (Berkeley: University of California Press, 1981), pp. 69–75.
12. E.g., *Nedarim* 66b.
13. *Sefer Hasidim*, no. 509.
14. *Iggeret HaKodesh* (Jerusalem, 1955). See now the English translation by Rabbi Seymour Cohen, *The Holy Letter* (New York: Ktav, 1976).
15. *Siddur Beit Ya'akov* (ed. Lemberg) pp. 135–61; *BCJL*, pp. 95–97, 100–103.
16. Rabbi Eliezer Berkowitz, *Crisis and Faith* (New York: Sanhedrin Press, 1976), pp. 48–82.

Chapter 8/Procreation

1. *Sefer HaHinnukh*, no. 1; *BCJL*, pp. 46ff.
2. Rabbi Meir Me'iri, *Torah Me'irah* (London, 1948), to Gen. 1:28.
3. *Tosafot* to *Bava Batra* 60b, s.v. *din hu.*
4. *Eduyot* I, 13; *Yevamot* 62a, b.
5. Noonan, op. cit., passim.
6. *Meshekh Hokhmah*, ad loc.
7. See *Shabbat* 119b and Midrash HaNe'elam Zohar Hadash to Gen. 2:3.
8. See J. David Bleich and Fred Rosner, eds., *Jewish Bioethics* (New York: Sanhedrin Press, 1979).
9. David M. Feldman, "Eugenics and Religious Law," in *Encyclopedia of Bioethics* (New York: Macmillan, 1978).
10. *Akedat Yitzhak*, to Gen., ad loc.
11. Viktor Aptowitzer, *Mavo L'Sefer Ravya*, p. 201.
12. Responsa *Naharei Afarsemon, Even HaEzer*, no. 18.
13. *Shir HaShirim Rabbah* I,4; *Pesikta d'Rav Kahana* XXII.

Chapter 9/This Matter of Abortion

1. *Sanhedrin* 72b; *BCJL*, chaps. 14 and 15.
2. Viktor Aptowitzer, "Observations on the Criminal Law of the Jews," *Jewish Quarterly Review* XV (1924), pp. 111ff.; *BCJL*, pp. 253–54.
3. Rashi; *Yad Ramah* to *Sanhedrin* 72b.
4. *BCJL*, p. 255.
5. *BCJL*, pp. 255–56.
6. *BCJL*, p. 258.
7. Aptowitzer, *JQR*, p. 88.

8. I. H. Weiss, *Dor Dor VeDor'shav* (1924), vol. II, p. 21.
9. Rabbi Isaac Schorr, Responsa *Koah Shor*, vol. I, no. 20 (dated 1755).
10. St. Fulgentius, *De Fide* 27, cited by E. Westermarck, *The Origin and Development of the Moral Ideas* (1908), vol. I, pp. 416–17. On use of the syringe in baptism, see H. W. Haggard, *Devils, Drugs and Doctors* (New York, 1929), p. 4.
11. *Sanhedrin* 110b; *Yalkut* to Psalms, no. 689.
12. See above, chap. 2.
13. *BCJL*, pp. 275 ff.
14. Rabbi I. Unterman, *Noam: A Volume for the Clarification of Halakhic Issues* (Hebrew), vol. VI (1963), p. 5; Rabbi I. Rosin, Responsa *Tzofenat Pa'aneah* (Dvinsk, 1934), no. 56.
15. Responsa *Mishpetei Uziel*, vol. III, *Hoshen Mishpat*, no. 47.
16. Responsa *Havvot Yair*, no. 31.
17. Responsa *Afarkasta D'Anya*, no. 169.
18. Responsa *Levushei Mordekhai, Hoshen Mishpat*, no. 139.
19. Responsa *Amud HaYemini*, no. 32 (1966) and Responsa *Tzitz Eliezer*, vol. IX, no. 51:3:9 (1967).

Chapter 10/Right to Life—Neonatal and Terminal

1. *Pesahim* 75a.
2. Isserles to *Tur* and to *Shulhan Arukh Yoreh Deah* 339:1.
3. Rabbi I. Jakobowitz, in *HaPardes* XXXI (1956), 1:28–31; *Jewish Medical Ethics* (New York: Bloch, 1975), pp. 121–25, 275–76.

Chapter 11/Aging, Death, and Afterlife

1. *The New York Times*, February 21, 1984, p. C–1.
2. *Yalkut Shimeoni*, no. 592.

Chapter 12/Moment of Death, Transplantation, and Autopsy

1. *Hakham Tzvi*, no. 77.
2. Responsa *Hatam Sofer, Yoreh Deah*, no. 338.
3. Rabbi I. Unterman, *Shevet MiYehudah*, vol. I, pp. 313ff.
4. *Noda BiYehudah, Yoreh Deah*, vol. II, no. 210.

Glossary of Hebrew Terms

Aggadah: As distinct from *Halakhah*, the nonlegal body of biblical interpretation.

Baraita: (See Talmud).

Bikkur Holim: The mitzvah of visiting the sick.

B'rit: Ritual circumcision.

Halakhah: Jewish law generally, or the specific legal ruling.

Kohen: Lit., "priest"; plural "*kohanim*." Descendants of Aaron who functioned in the sanctuary and later retained priestly privileges and restrictions.

Midrash: Lit., "exposition," an extra-talmudic recension of interpretation to the Bible, both halakhic and aggadic.

Mishnah: (See Talmud).

Mishneh Torah: The codification of all of Jewish law by Maimonides (1135–1204). Set forth in fourteen books, it is also known as *Yad* (= 14) *HaHazakah*, or *Yad*.

Mitzvah: Lit., a commandment, an obligation. By extension, a meritorious deed.

Nefesh: A soul; a person.

Onah: Conjugal relations.

Pikkuah Nefesh: Lit., "life saving." A situation where life or health are threatened.

Rashi: Rabbi Solomon Yitzhaki (d. 1105). The commentator *par excellence* on Bible and Talmud.

Sanhedrin: The high court.

Shulhan Arukh: Lit., "The Set Table," the codification of applicable Jewish Law by Joseph Karo (d. 1575). Printed with the "Tablecloth," the Glosses, of Moses Isserles (d. 1572) to add Ashkenazi legal tradition to that of Spanish-Portuguese and Mediterranean. (Sefardic). The *Kitzur Shulhan Arukh* is a brief handbook of everyday procedures, composed by Rabbi Solomon Ganzfried in 1863.

Talmud: The library of legal and extralegal commentary to and application of biblical law and narrative. Its fundamental layer is the *Mishnah*, redacted about 200 C.E., formulating the laws of the Oral Tradition and more. Discussion and elaboration of the Mishnah—and of other contemporaneous literary traditions, such as *Baraita*—are called *G'mara*, and all together are called Talmud. The Talmud's main recension is the Babylonian one, Talmud Bavli, emanating from the academies there and concluding its deliberations about 500 C.E. A parallel development took place in the academies of Palestine, coming to a close a century earlier. The Babylonian Talmud is far more exhaustive than the Palestinian one, and predominated in Jewish history as the object of intensive study and the reigning authority in Jewish law. Legal norms are also derivable from its commentators, such as Rashi's explanatory glosses, or the critical analyses of *Tosafot*, the scholars of medieval France and environs. These are, in fact, printed alongside the text in published editions of the Talmud.

Torah: Lit., "teaching." In the narrow sense, the Five Books of Moses; in the wider sense, all of scripture and commentaries; by extension, the sum of Jewish religious teaching and tradition.